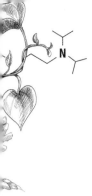
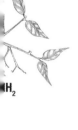
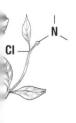

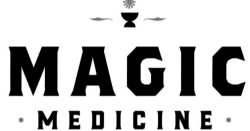

MAGIC
· MEDICINE ·

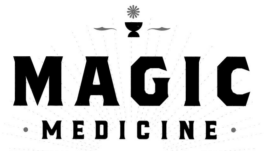

MAGIC
· MEDICINE ·

A TRIP THROUGH
THE INTOXICATING HISTORY
AND

**MODERN-DAY USE
OF PSYCHEDELIC PLANTS
&
SUBSTANCES**

CODY JOHNSON

FAIR WINDS

First Published in 2018 by Fair Winds Press, an imprint of The Quarto Group,
100 Cummings Center, Suite 265-D, Beverly, MA 01915, USA.
T (978) 282-9590 F (978) 283-2742 QuartoKnows.com

Fair Winds Press titles are also available at discount for retail, wholesale, promotional, and bulk purchase. For details, contact the Special Sales Manager by email at specialsales@quarto.com or by mail at The Quarto Group, Attn: Special Sales Manager, 100 Cummings Center, Suite 265-D, Beverly, MA 01915, USA.

23   6

ISBN: 978-1-59233-772-9

Digital edition published in 2018
eISBN: 978-1-63159-428-1

Library of Congress Cataloging-in-Publication Data is available

Design: Landers Miller Design
Cover Design: Landers Miller Design
Illustrations: Holly Neel

Printed in China

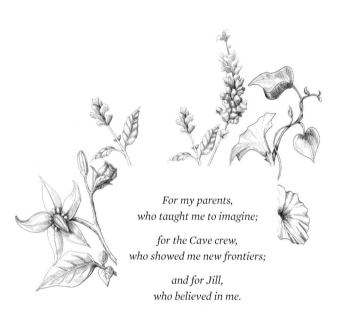

For my parents,
who taught me to imagine;

for the Cave crew,
who showed me new frontiers;

and for Jill,
who believed in me.

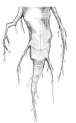

CONTENTS

18–113

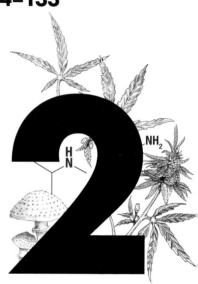

114–133

1 CLASSICAL PSYCHEDELICS

2 EMPATHOGENIC PSYCHEDELICS

134–171

172–223

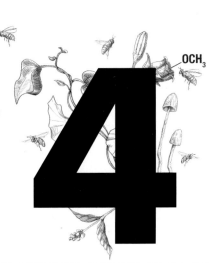

DISSOCIATIVE PSYCHEDELICS

UNIQUE PSYCHEDELICS

A PEEK INTO THE FUTURE

OF

PSYCHEDELIC MEDICINE

It's Tuesday morning, and you wander into your local Psychedelic Clinic. At the front desk they take your name: "Yes," says the receptionist, "we're expecting you. Right this way." You're whisked into a comfortable room where an open window bathes a wall of bookshelves in yellow light.

The therapist enters, but looks more like a neighborly professor—horn-rim glasses, brown vest, a pair of loafers. "Have a seat," he says, nodding toward a cozy-looking couch. He hands you a glass of water and a small pill containing 150 milligrams of pure MDMA (Ecstasy). You take it and lean back. The session begins.

Sound absurd? If advocates of psychedelic-assisted therapy get their way, this scene might not be that far-fetched. Rick Doblin, founder and executive director of MAPS—the Multidisciplinary Association for Psychedelic Studies, a nonprofit dedicated to researching psychedelics—estimates that MDMA therapy will be approved by the U.S. Food and Drug Administration (FDA) by 2021. After decades on the front lines of advocacy and research, MAPS is on the cusp of pushing the very first psychedelic into the realm of accepted medicine.

And, if the swarm of recent publications on the benefits of psilocybin, LSD, and ayahuasca are any indication, MDMA is merely the first domino to fall. With the scientific evidence mounting in favor of therapeutic use for these once-feared substances, a world in which special clinics offer compassionate guidance for mental, emotional, and even spiritual development with psychedelics is beginning to seem less like a dream and more like an inevitability.

ARE YOU EXPERIENCED?

It all starts, of course, with the psychedelic experience. To anyone familiar with them, psychedelics need no description. Indeed, words could never capture the bizarre, dimension-bending, and profoundly emotional worlds they unlock. The very prospect is laughable. How could you wrangle something as elusive as consciousness into a net as crude as human language?

To adapt a famous quip credited to Martin Mull, writing about psychedelics is like dancing about architecture. But this particular dance remains compelling— in spite of the apparent futility, trippers 'round the world keep sharing stories of their psychedelic experiences on the Internet, while hungry readers, some equally adventurous, others only vicariously so, follow along, spellbound, from faraway reaches of the globe.

Having found the standard lexicon wanting, psychedelic enthusiasts have developed their own lingo for these hard-to-pin-down effects. Everyone knows "trippy," a generic term that applies to anything that resembles the perception-bending effects of psychedelics, whether an echoing guitar riff or a fractal-based poster. Online "trip reports"—first-person accounts of psychedelic experiences, including details on dosage, intensity, and duration—often feature descriptions of a molecule's "headspace" and "body load." Headspace refers to the sum of mental effects: the overall mood and state of cognition a psychedelic produces. Body load, however, is used to describe unpleasant physical sensations, such as heaviness and constriction. There's even a word for these psychedelic explorers—"psychonauts," derived from the Greek roots for *soul* and *voyager*.

We are fascinated, even the sworn-sober teetotalers among us, by altered states of consciousness and the plants and chemicals that unlock them. That so little material —a handful of leaves, a pinch of white powder—could induce in us such fundamental and overwhelming changes is awesome and more than a little humbling.

Psychedelics dissolve boundaries—both within human beings and between them. Bridging seemingly irreconcilable gaps, the story of psychedelics brings together science and religion, art and philosophy, botany and pharmaceutical engineering, and modern medicine and ancient shamanism. Because the psychedelic experience is, at root, a deeply human experience, there is little it does not touch.

THE REAL RISKS

Wherever they grow, throughout history and in most traditional cultures, psyche-delic plants and fungi have been revered as sacraments and powerful medicines. Yet, the attitude of modern Western culture toward these astounding organisms is dismissive, prohibitive, and even fearful—we must destroy what we do not under-stand. This approach stands in stark contrast to the many indigenous peoples who have learned to integrate psychedelics into their life journeys, passing the sacred knowledge of their proper usage from generation to generation. It also contrasts with the evidence that suggests the classical psychedelics are among the least harmful of all "abused" substances. No overdose deaths from LSD, psilocybin, or peyote have ever been recorded. A number of deaths and injuries have resulted from reckless behavior, including mixing psychedelics with other drugs, taking excessive doses without supervision, and tripping while driving or hiking, but these can be avoided with proper preparation and education. As clinical research attests, using psychedelics under controlled conditions is remarkably safe.

The dark irony of our culture's stance toward these "dangerous" chemicals is that by prohibiting them, we have only amplified their dangers. When people buy "Ecstasy" or "Molly," they don't know what they're getting or how much. Imagine ordering a martini at a bar and not knowing whether you'll receive a martini or a triple shot of high-proof grain liquor—or a concoction with no alcohol, but a potent blend of caffeine, ketamine, methamphetamine, and stimulants you've never heard of. That's the situation with all illicit psychedelic substances. And users who find themselves in a medical crisis are often reluctant to seek help for fear of incriminating themselves. Far from reducing the harms associated with psychedelics, the prohibitive approach actually maximizes their risks. To truly address the risks of psychedelic use would require a swift about-face in public policy, focusing on regulation and education rather than punitive measures that brand psychedelic users as felons.

Among shamans, psychedelic substances are often called "teacher plants," a reminder that the experience is not sought for its own sake but always to learn. For them, the psychedelic experience is the furthest thing from recreational—a healing journey, a vision quest, and a rite of passage, yes, but no Saturday night bender. In our Western culture, where the War on Drugs rages on, the distinction is rarely made between visionary substances and addictive vices such as heroin and methamphetamine. It doesn't help that psychedelics carry all the baggage of the 1960s, and, for many, still symbolize the reckless hedonism of that era.

Yet, their "unauthorized" use remains widely popular. In thatched huts in the deepest reaches of the Amazon rainforest, at Burning Man in the middle of Nevada's scorching Black Rock Desert, at electronic music festivals and nightclubs, on therapists' couches, and beneath the stars—almost anywhere there are people, there are people taking psychedelics.

A PSYCHEDELIC BY ANY OTHER NAME

What exactly is a psychedelic, anyway? The term "psychedelic" is a relatively new one, having emerged in the 1950s in correspondence between two intellectuals of the age. Fascinated by the relatively new compound LSD, as well as its age-old cactus-derived cousin mescaline, the writer Aldous Huxley and the psychiatrist and researcher Humphry Osmond sought to coin a term that would encapsulate the unique effects of these substances.

LSD and mescaline had previously been classed as "psychotomimetic"— literally, "imitating insanity"—or as "hallucinogens," which reduces these complex compounds to a single symptom. Neither was satisfactory. Eventually, Osmond suggested "psychedelic," from the Greek roots for "mind manifesting." The rest is history. Today, just about everyone, from psychologists and chemists to artists and musicians, understands "psychedelic" to mean those trippy molecules that turn our perception of the world—and of ourselves—on its head.

But the borders of its definition are fuzzy. Sometimes, the word is used to indicate only the "classical" psychedelics, which act at serotonin receptors: LSD, psilocybin, mescaline, and their ilk. The term can be expanded to include four separate classes of substance:

1. The aforementioned serotonin-oriented compounds, of which there are hundreds
2. "Dissociatives," such as ketamine and salvia, which produce the sensation of detachment from one's body
3. "Empathogens," such as MDMA, which, although less overtly "trippy" than other substances, still amplify emotions and insights in a decidedly psychedelic way
4. "Unique" substances that can't easily be categorized, including cannabinoids such as THC, which, in high doses, can induce visionary reveries

The so-called deliriants, such as deadly nightshade and datura, are typically excluded. Though unquestionably hallucinogenic, deliriants are so different from traditional psychedelics—and so unpleasant—they're usually classed separately.

In this book, I take the broad view, including all major psychedelics, a few dissociatives and empathogens, and a couple borderline deliriants. They all share one major quality: rather than simply amplifying familiar aspects of consciousness, such as pleasure, psychedelic drugs produce unique states of being unavailable during waking consciousness and utterly alien to the sober mind.

Anyone who has ever wondered about psychedelics—from complete neophytes to veteran trippers, seekers and sages to skeptics and scientists, therapists and patients to green thumbs and armchair anthropologists—will find something here. Each chapter dives into the rich history of a single plant or compound and explores its therapeutic and spiritual uses—not only in indigenous contexts, but in modern medicine where psychedelics are quickly earning a reputation as powerful healing agents. Finally, each chapter is sprinkled with firsthand quotes which attempt to pry open the "doors of perception," allowing glimmers of psychedelic light to fall upon sober minds.

Among so many cultures, the ritual use of psychedelics is a deeply embedded cultural institution, helping people connect to their ancestors, their gods, and themselves in a way that no other tool allows. Anyone interested in the condition of humankind—complex, emotive, and painfully self-aware, conscious of the past but peering into an uncertain future, always asking questions and assembling new stories about the world we inhabit—should be curious about psychedelics.

This book is not stuffy and academic. No background in botany, chemistry, or medicine is necessary—come as you are and learn about some of the most fascinating plants and molecules on the planet. Nor is this an instruction manual—for information on how to use these substances, readers will have to look elsewhere.

Within these pages you'll find ayahuasca, the acrid jungle potion wrought from the synergy of two plants—either of which would be completely ineffective without the other. Though it has served as the visionary pillar of Amazonian shamanism for millennia, word has gotten out, and "spiritual tourists" now flock to Peru in the hopes of finding themselves at the bottom of a bitter clay cup.

Ayahuasca's main psychoactive component, DMT, has become famous in its own right. Removed from its native context and vaporized by enterprising mental voyagers, DMT offers most users a 15-minute rocket ship to alien dimensions. According to many users, these surreal inner landscapes are peopled with otherworldly creatures and other "DMT entities" who perform impossible acts of magic for their astounded human visitors.

Then, there's DiPT, a little-known but unique compound. Whereas most psychedelics are famous for their swirling visual hallucinations, DiPT distorts the perception of sounds, lowering everything in pitch like a helium balloon in reverse. Whether it renders music heavenly or diabolic depends on whom you ask.

The usual suspects make an appearance, of course: LSD, perhaps the most famous mind-altering substance of the twentieth century; psilocybin, the "magic" in magic mushrooms; and peyote, the slow-growing cactus revered by the natives of Mexico's Chihuahuan Desert.

There's also "mad honey"—an exotic Himalayan nectar produced by cliff-dwelling bees, rich with psychoactive compounds sourced from the rhododendron flowers that dot the hillsides. And ketamine, the go-to for anesthesiologists, clubbers, and astral travelers alike, which is now being investigated for its incredible antidepressant effects. And that's just the beginning—nature's bounteous pharmacy extends to psychedelic frogs, fish, and even sea sponges.

You'll also find a cast of colorful characters, from Sir Humphry Davy—a brilliant nineteenth-century chemist who inhaled so much nitrous oxide it nearly killed him—to Alexander Shulgin—the godfather of psychedelic chemistry, a modern-day molecular wizard who discovered hundreds of new synthetic psychedelics and popularized MDMA, or Ecstasy.

Along the way, you'll encounter Timothy Leary, the Harvard professor-turned-countercultural-guru who coined the phrase, "Turn on, tune in, drop out;" Ken Kesey, the author and leader of the Merry Pranksters; John C. Lilly, the controversial researcher who studied dolphins, language, and psychedelics, sometimes all at once; and Terence McKenna, the bard from the beyond who waxed poetic about alien intelligence, heroic doses, and stoned apes.

After a decades-long hiatus—thanks to the enactment of the War on Drugs in the wake of the turbulent 1960s—psychedelic research is officially back. Only this time, instead of arriving with longhaired hippies in the countercultural van, it's coming by way of soft-talking therapists and white-coated neuroscientists. First psychedelic music and art, now psychedelic science and medicine—bit by bit, psychedelics are becoming mainstream.

It's not that the laws have changed—drug prohibition still presents numerous roadblocks to this kind of research—but, today, there are many more scientists willing to jump the bureaucratic hurdles to study psychedelics.

Government agencies are also beginning to warm up to these once-forbidden fruits. MAPS, the nonprofit spearheading most psychedelic research in the United States, is collaborating with the FDA to investigate MDMA with the aim of regulating it as a prescription drug for post-traumatic stress disorder. MAPS has also collaborated with the U. S. Department of Veterans Affairs to study whether MDMA-assisted therapy can help soldiers recover from trauma.

In recent years, psychedelics have shown promise in treating a remarkable array of mental conditions, including depression, obsessive-compulsive disorder, end-of-life anxiety, cluster headaches, and even substance addiction. Each new study serves to vindicate the age-old claims of indigenous peoples—that these substances are, in fact, powerful healing medicines.

When administered to dying patients suffering from treatment-resistant anxiety, psilocybin and LSD demonstrate an astonishing effect. After a single session, a majority of participants found their fears dissolved. They came to terms with their mortality, enabling them to live their remaining days in fullness and peace.

Psychedelics may harbor good news for people looking to kick their habit. LSD has been shown to reduce problem drinking in alcoholics, and psilocybin has demonstrated early promise as an aid to quitting cigarettes. Ibogaine, a unique psychedelic derived from an African shrub, has gained such momentum among heroin addicts that ibogaine rehab clinics are popping up around the world.

Ketamine, too, has emerged as a promising substance for mental illnesses. Strictly speaking a dissociative and not a psychedelic (but included in this book, using the broader definition of "psychedelic"), ketamine has been used to treat alcoholism, opioid addiction, chronic pain, and, especially, major depression. Even the most untreatable cases of depression often react favorably to an injection of ketamine, with mood-stabilizing effects lasting for about one week. Though the science is young, ketamine therapy clinics have already sprung up in the United States.

The common worry that psychedelics are dangerous for mental health is mostly unfounded. Two recent studies determined there was no relationship between psychedelic use and mental health problems. In fact, psychedelics appeared to exhibit a protective effect: People who had used them reported lower psychological distress and fewer suicide attempts. In a separate study, prisoners who had used psychedelics were less likely to return to jail than any other groups of prisoners—including their non-drug-using counterparts.

Beyond turning modern psychiatry on its head, psychedelics are also spurring advances in neuroscience. At London's Imperial College, researchers have taken the first ever brain scans of human beings on LSD and psilocybin. The results were surprising. The tripping brain is not hyperactive, as one would think, but it is more chaotic and more creative than the sober brain, enabling, what one neuroscientist termed "a state of unconstrained cognition."

Psychedelics interest neuroscientists for the same reason they interest shamans, artists, and mental explorers: They fundamentally perturb consciousness, the very core of our being, thus telling us more about ourselves. As Dr. David Nutt, a leader in psychedelic neuroscience research, put it: "If you want to understand consciousness, you've got to study psychedelics."

Scientific understanding is finally catching up to the shamans and medicine men who have sworn by these substances for ages. Truly, there has never been a more exciting time for psychedelic science, medicine, and spirituality. As fascinating as the history of these plants and substances may be, the future promises to be even brighter.

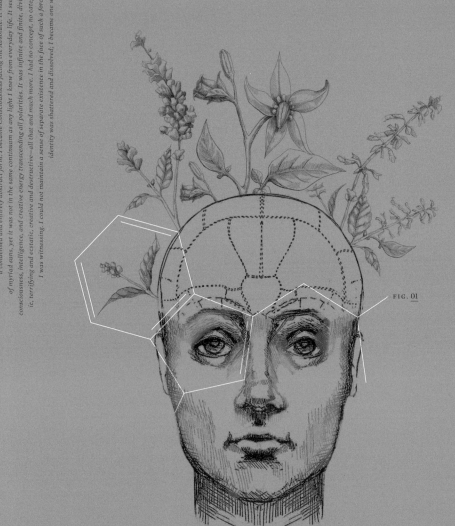

My entity was a mass of human swirling on... of... immense proportions that as I... to contain all of Existence, a condensed and entirely abstract form. I became Consciousness facing the Absolute. It had the brig... of myriad suns, yet it was not in the same continuum as any light I knew from everyday life. It seemed to... consciousness, intelligence, and creative energy transcending all polarities. It was infinite and finite, divine and... ie, terrifying and ecstatic, creative and destructive—all that and much more. I had no concept, no categories for... I was witnessing. I could not maintain a sense of separate existence in the face of such a force. My ow... identity was shattered and dissolved; I became one with the S...

FIG. 01

CHAPTER ONE

CLASSICAL PSYCHEDELICS

From time-honored shamanic tools to brand new molecular inventions, the classical psychedelics elicit their effects by tickling the brain's serotonin system. Including such iconic substances as LSD, psilocybin mushrooms, and peyote cacti, this collection defines what it means to be psychedelic.

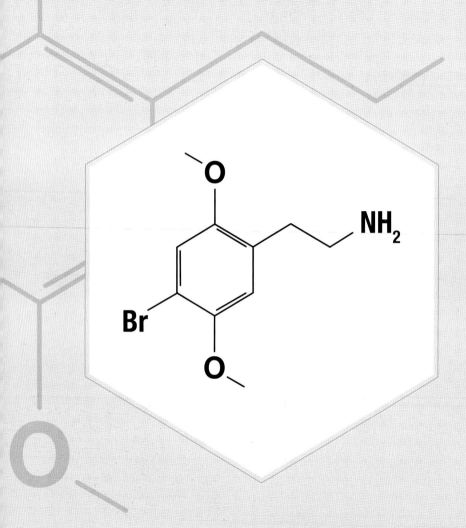

FIG. 1.1

2-(4-BROMO-2,5-DIMETHOXYPHENYL) ETHYLAMINE

2C-B AND
THE 2C FAMILY

ASSOCIATED WITH *underground psychotherapy and the modern psychedelic scene*

ORIGINS AND BACKGROUND

THE STORY OF THE 2C FAMILY OF CHEMICALS BEGINS IN 1974 with one man, but spans decades and has touched the lives of many thousands. What began as an offhand experiment by an eccentric chemist would soon yield some of the most significant psychedelic molecules of the modern era.

When the eminent psychedelic chemist Alexander Shulgin and his colleague Michael Carter debuted 2C-B in 1975, they could not have known the beast they were unleashing. This chemical would spawn a series of related compounds whose merits and shortcomings would be hotly discussed by chemists, therapists, and consciousness explorers for decades.

Whether on a rave dance floor or the therapist's couch, 2C-B and its ilk spelled upheaval. Agents of change are always feared, however, and it's no surprise most of these compounds were soon outlawed in many countries —even though their therapeutic potential appeared to outweigh their relatively low toxicity. Once widely available in Amsterdam head shops and online marketplaces, most of the 2C compounds are now relegated to the black market.

Members of the 2C series count among Shulgin's most popular creations, including the lucid aphrodisiac 2C-B. He was especially proud of them, and, by most accounts, rightfully so.

In the early 1970s, Shulgin was experimenting with DOB, an "extremely potent and long-lived" psychedelic amphetamine he'd found seven years earlier, when he discovered the 2C series. Shulgin realized that, with a single tweak, every member of the "DOx" family could yield a potent 2C derivative. And *voilà*—a whole new series of chemicals was born, each with its own psychoactive profile.

To name each new compound, Shulgin used the final letter of its prototype: 2C-B is based on DOB, 2C-I is based on DOI, and so on. All the 2C chemicals are identical to their namesakes, except for that one inspired tweak first made by a chemical wizard back in the 1970s.

ALEXANDER SHULGIN, THE PSYCHEDELIC CHEMIST

The story of psychedelic chemistry is, in large part, the story of Alexander "Sasha" Shulgin, the prolific chemist who designed and popularized so many of these drugs. An elder statesman of the psychedelic community and a perennial tinkerer of both mind and matter, Shulgin dedicated his life to discovering, synthesizing, and personally testing hundreds of novel psychoactive drugs.

In a career lasting more than a half century, he almost single-handedly developed the field of psychedelic chemistry while pushing it to new frontiers. By the time he died in 2014 at the age of eighty-eight, he was a celebrated icon among psychedelic enthusiasts.

Sasha and his wife, Ann—a psychedelic therapist, speaker, and author in her own right—frequently sampled new compounds from Sasha's lab. They were adventurous, but not careless: Sasha always started with miniscule doses before graduating to larger amounts and insisted on being the first tester in case a new substance proved toxic or unpleasant.

Sasha's interest in psychedelics began in the late 1950s when he first tried mescaline. He enjoyed a successful career at Dow Chemical, but his passion remained with the mysterious mental catalysts he'd sampled earlier. Ann once estimated her husband had tripped about four thousand times in his life—that's more than once a week for over forty years!

Sasha prized the special experience of first contact. Like world explorers centuries before him, Shulgin voyaged far from home and planted the first flags on many new geographies of consciousness—the epitome of the term "psychonaut," or consciousness explorer. Rather than mighty wooden ships, the chemist launched himself with the tiniest amounts of colorless powders. Though his destination was uncertain, the excitement was palpable: He felt an "incredible tingle" every time he synthesized some molecule never before seen on Earth—"and I'll be the first to know what it does."

Whenever a compound proved worthy of further analysis, the Shulgins would share it with a group of close friends. This informal research group would test the new chemical at different doses and report back on its duration, psychedelic qualities, and other effects.

At the same time, Sasha fostered an unlikely alliance with the U. S. Drug Enforcement Administration (DEA). As a special consultant, he educated the agents on novel substances, provided drug samples, and occasionally served as an expert witness in court. In return, he was granted a Schedule I license— essentially carte blanche to produce chemicals that would otherwise risk hefty jail sentences. The personal lab he set up behind his house outside Berkeley, California, would be the envy of any clandestine chemist: With unrestricted access to rare chemical precursors and the ability to produce new and banned chemicals without risk of arrest, he was truly a free agent.

But the chemist's partnership with the DEA would not last forever. The Shulgins believed information about drugs belonged to everybody, not just law enforcement. In 1991, they published the results of their personal research in a groundbreaking volume called *PiHKAL (Phenethylamines I Have Known and Loved): A Chemical Love Story*. The book was split into two parts: half autobiography, detailing the couple's personal love story; and half cookbook, with step-by-step synthesis instructions and subjective impressions of each substance's effects. The DEA wasn't happy with the publication. They clamped down on Shulgin's lab and asked him to turn in his Schedule I license as payback.

Undeterred, Sasha continued producing and testing new compounds. In 1997, the Shulgins published another eight hundred-page tome, *TiHKAL*, the tryptamines equivalent of its predecessor. The tryptamine chemical family includes LSD, DMT, and psilocybin; the phenethylamines include mescaline, MDMA, and 2C-B. Together, the books covered more than two hundred chemicals in detail, while briefly touching on hundreds more.

The influence of these books, together with Shulgin's many scientific papers, cannot be overstated. He was an open-source chemist, freely sharing the synthesis steps for the hundreds of new compounds he created. His methods focused on easily obtainable precursors, presumably to help underground chemists replicate his work.

For decades, chemists, drug users, legislators, and law enforcement officials kept a close eye as new compounds churned out of Sasha's lab. Within weeks of publishing the chemical synthesis for a new compound, it would appear for sale online, often produced by a gray-market lab in China. And then, of course, the DEA would ban it, and a new breed of chemicals would emerge, often inspired by another Shulgin publication.

THE EXPERIENCE

Of all of Shulgin's inventions, 2C-B stands apart. The first and most famous of the 2Cs, it has earned praise as a superlative psychedelic, frequently mentioned in the same breath as mescaline and LSD. Lucid, gentle, and even erotic, 2C-B has been celebrated by generations of psychonauts for its aesthetic beauty and manageability. A remarkably flexible compound, it is easily molded to the user's intentions, especially at low to moderate doses.

Where some psychedelics can be extremely stimulating and tie the tongue into knots, 2C-B is relatively calm and leaves one's communication faculties largely intact. When someone is teetering on the precipice of a drug-induced mental crisis, grasping at any rope that leads back to reality, the ability to communicate can mean the difference between momentary anxiety and a full-fledged freak-out. Among the mildest and shortest of psychedelic experiences, 2C-B often serves as a tripper's first encounter with psychedelics.

Shulgin considered 2C-B his favorite of all substances. He took it often, referring to it as the "Great Teacher." Perhaps more than any other drug, 2C-B has been celebrated for its sensual nature. One of Shulgin's testers gave this report:

> The love-making was phenomenal, passionate, ecstatic, lyric, animal, loving, tender, sublime . . . I am aware of every muscle and nerve in my body, unbelievably erotic, quiet and exquisite, almost unbearable.

In a 2003 column for the Center for Cognitive Liberty & Ethics, Sasha extolled 2C-B's virtues as:

> One of the most graceful, erotic, sensual, introspective compounds I have ever invented. For most people, it is a short-lived and comfortable psychedelic, with neither toxic side-effects nor next-day hang-over. Its effects are felt very much in the body, as well as in the mind . . . 2C-B opens up the emotional, intuitive and archetypal area of your psyche to help you solve [your problems].

A BROAD APPEAL

Indeed, 2C-B originally gained popularity among therapists and their patients who found the compound very effective at fostering compassionate relationships and bringing traumas and insecurities to light in a nonthreatening way. As with MDMA, however, word got out and 2C-B quickly expanded beyond its therapeutic roots. The compound invaded dance floors and bedrooms as it gained renown as a tactile, emotional, and sexual enhancer. During its legal heyday, a German company even marketed it as an aphrodisiac called Erox.

Dutch "smart shops" also sold 2C-B as an Ecstasy-like legal high under the name "Nexus." That moniker is still used occasionally, and it's especially fitting for a substance at the intersection of so many interests and disciplines. From chemistry and psychiatry to music and romance, 2C-B crosses many paths.

When politics and law enforcement joined the ranks of those interested in 2C-B, its days as a legal high were numbered. The United States banned it in 1995; by 2000, it was prohibited around the world.

By meaning many things to many people, 2C-B illuminates the arbitrary nature of our labels for drugs. Where therapists saw a remarkable new medicine, couples found a powerful aphrodisiac and young ravers found a hip new flavor of consciousness to tap into. Meanwhile, law enforcement agencies and many well-meaning but poorly informed citizens—egged on by sensational media reports and decades of antidrug propaganda—saw, and continue to see, only a dangerous club drug. 2C-B is all of these, and yet none. The molecule remains the same; only our approach to it changes.

THE COUSINS: 2C-E, 2C-I, AND 2C-C

For the most part, the other 2C chemicals—and there are dozens, if not hundreds—are variations on a theme. All share certain qualities, including "trippy" head-space, unusual bodily sensations, and seemingly "digitized" psychedelic visual distortions. Yet each one offers a distinct flavor.

2C-E is notorious for its intensity. Even seasoned trippers describe it as a challenging substance, producing deep and introspective mental states that can catch the unwary traveler by surprise. It's often described as a "cold teacher," but one with valuable lessons. The physical sensations, including tingling pins and needles that cover the entire body, can be overwhelming. For some serious explorers, however, the rewards justify the journey. 2C-E's fans say it offers unparalleled personal insights and exceptional visual effects.

2C-I and 2C-C are somewhat lighter fare and more often used in recreational contexts. They last about four to seven hours. Visuals tend towards fractals, and the headspace is said to be trippy but not overwhelming at typical doses. Still, the margin of error is small—a few milligrams can spell the difference between an amusing night out and a psychic meltdown. The bodily sensations can also be intense, especially with 2C-I. What some people call an incredible sense of tactile energy is, for others, an uncomfortable "body load" which only the passage of time can relieve.

THE FUTURE OF 2C-B IN PSYCHEDELIC THERAPY

Perhaps it's not truly the end for psychedelic therapy, but rather a very slow and bumpy beginning. MDMA is now back in the limelight, having returned to its roots as a therapeutic tool of great interest to psychiatry (see pages 125 to 133). LSD and psilocybin are once again emerging as legitimate medicines for conditions ranging from anxiety to tobacco addiction (see pages 70 to 73 and 97 to 101). Maybe someday, the 2C chemicals, beloved by therapists, lovers, African healers, and ravers alike, will emerge from the darkness into the realm of legal medicines. If they do, it will likely be 2C-B leading the charge.

MEDICINE OF THE SINGING ANCESTORS

In South Africa, the *sangomas*, or medicine men, of the Xhosa people traditionally used a variety of local plants to produce a visionary brew they would consume at tribal ceremonies. Called *Ubulawu Nomathotholo*, or "medicine of the singing ancestors," the shamans would consume this foamy concoction to facilitate healing, prophesying, and communicating with ancestors. *Ubulawu* had long been a cornerstone of the Xhosa way of life.

But because of the increasing rarity and expense of these visionary plants and their considerable toxicity, the *sangomas* began using 2C-B as a surrogate. While it was legal in the 1990s, the healers obtained the substance from local herbal shops who imported it from abroad.

To the Xhosa healers, 2C-B served as a worthy substitute, even surpassing their traditional plant-based potion in some regards. It was easily accessible, physically comfortable, and had very few negative side effects. Most important, the *sangomas* were pleased to discover it took them to the same spirit realm as their traditional medicines. But it wasn't to last: The new *Ubulawu* was banned in 1998, and Xhosa shamans have had to make do with rarer and more toxic plant substances ever since.

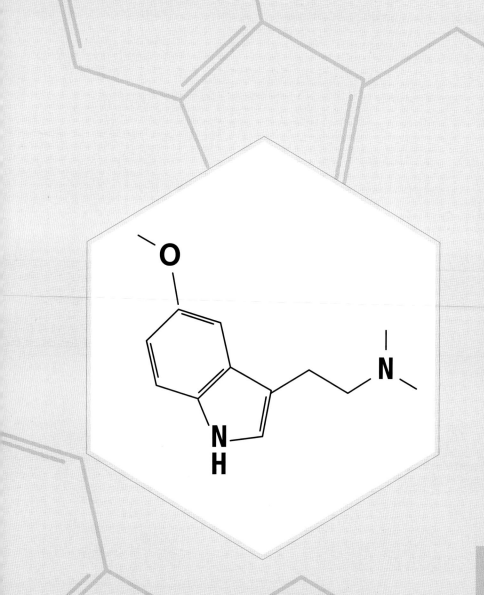

FIG. 1.2

5-METHOXY-*N*,*N*-DIMETHYLTRYPTAMINE

DISCOVERED

Used since antiquity; first
synthesized in 1936; first
identified in plants in
1959; first identified in
toad venom in 1965

5-MEO-DMT

DURATION

5 to 20 minutes vaporized;
1 to 3 hours insufflated
(sniffed)

ASSOCIATED WITH *indigenous peoples in the western Amazon basin*

ORIGINS AND BACKGROUND

5-MEO-DMT IS AS DIVERSE AND ENIGMATIC AS ONE substance can be. It is one of humanity's oldest sacraments, yet one of our newest discoveries. It provides an overwhelming, profound, and sacred experience, yet it is used casually by men of the Yanomami tribes on a daily basis. It is both rare and exceptionally common—though it occurs naturally in dozens of plants and animals, including humans, the chemical remains obscure and is rarely encountered on the underground drug market. And it is both organic and synthetic—once the exclusive product of nature, concentrated in especially high quantities in the bark of certain jungle trees, it is now easily manufactured in labs around the world.

The bow on this package of paradoxes was tied in 1965, when high levels of 5-MeO-DMT were identified in the venom of the Colorado River Toad. This discovery holds more significance than it sounds—although the plant world teems with psychedelic molecules, animals with high quantities of such substances are practically unheard of. The toad appears to be unique, though many of its relatives in the *Bufo* genus produce bufotenine, only the Colorado River Toad, *Bufo alvarius*, bears an enzyme that converts it into plentiful 5-MeO-DMT.

Some people have taken to "milking" the venom from the toads' parotid glands and vaporizing it for psychedelic effects. Animal lovers may take some solace: This is said to be painless, involving nothing more than a glass slide rubbed against the toad's glands to collect the goo. In some areas, however, the toad is classified as a threatened species and may not be removed from its habitat legally. Some media outlets have sensationalized "toad licking" as a new phenomenon, but these reports are probably exaggerated if not outright false. Because the venom contains other toxins, which appear to be destroyed by heat when vaporized, leaving only the desired compounds intact—direct consumption by licking is ill advised. As bizarre as it sounds, smoking toad venom marks a pioneering step for humanity: Along with "mad" honey and certain species of visionary fish, it is one of the only psychedelic experiences sourced from animals.

CLOSER TO HOME

5-MeO-DMT is not just an elusive jungle potion, limited to a few shamans and adventurous toad smokers. Within ten years of the toad discovery, science threw another curveball: several studies confirmed the existence of 5-MeO-DMT in human tissues. It is still one of only two known "endogenous" entheogens—psychedelics produced naturally by the human body. The other is N,N-DMT—often shortened to DMT—and the exact function of both remains a mystery.

Once considered exotic and obscure, 5-MeO-DMT turns out to be surprisingly widespread: Every one of us is a walking supply closet. This leads to a few awkward questions—as DMT and 5-MeO-DMT are illegal, does that make our bodies contraband? Technically, yes. Legislators haven't bothered to address that conundrum, and, until they do, you could, within the letter of the law, be booked for possession of a controlled substance. Someone needs to bring attention to this loophole, but the airport security line is probably not the best place to do it.

5-MeO-DMT may be little known outside select circles, but it packs a punch that far exceeds its small reputation. Structurally related to DMT—often considered the most powerful of all psychedelics—the 5-MeO variant is said to be even more overwhelming. Proponents insist its ability to launch users to a spiritual state of oneness is unparalleled. Wade Davis, an anthropologist who studied the Yanomami people, compared the epená snuff ritual to "being shot out of a rifle barrel lined with Baroque paintings and landing on a sea of electricity."

EPENÁ, A SPIRITUAL SNUFF FROM SOUTH AMERICA

Traces of 5-MeO-DMT have been identified in archaeological artifacts that date back thousands of years. Though urban psychonauts today usually vaporize the isolated chemical from a glass pipe, historically, it has been consumed as part of a plant-based snuff.

In the traditional method, a shaman uses a hollowed-out bone as a pipe to forcibly blow the snuff into the recipient's nostrils, where it is absorbed through the mucus membranes. This process produces a longer, less intense experience than vaporizing and inhaling the substance, but it also leaves a burning sensation in the nasal passages. Some tribes also eat the snuff in the form of pellets, absorbing the active compounds through the gut.

The snuffs are made primarily from *Virola* trees, a genus in the nutmeg family whose bark resins are rich in 5-MeO-DMT. Although *Virola* trees grow all over South America, only tribes in the north-western Amazon and Orinoco basins seem to have discovered the secrets contained in their bark. To prepare the snuff, the shaman heats the bark and scrapes the amber resin into a pot, boils it down to a thick syrup, and leaves it to dry in the sun. The resulting red-brown condensed resin is ground to a very fine powder—known as epená, or "semen of the sun."

Among the Yanomami tribes along the border between Brazil and Venezuela, epená is prized as both sacrament and casual intoxicant. During ceremonies, Yanomami shamans take very heavy doses to enter a trance state, chanting and singing to invite contact with small mountain spirits called *hekura*. Hekura are usually sought for their healing powers, though they are also said to endow shamans with abilities such as instantaneous transport across great distances. Once a hekura has taken residence in his body, the shaman can call on its curative and other magical powers.

Its intensity is matched by its potency—at roughly five times the strength of DMT, you certainly would not want to confuse the two. When vaporized, it is active as low as 2 milligrams; 10 milligrams is enough to skyrocket most people to another dimension. As one user writes: "If most hallucinogens, including LSD, merely distort reality, however bizarrely, 5-MeO-DMT completely dissolves reality as we know it, leaving neither hallucinations nor anyone to watch them. The experience . . . is not for the novice."

The effects are said to be ineffable, but that hasn't stopped countless explorers from attempting to describe them. As with DMT, online "trip reports" often mention its sudden and extreme intensity, with the onset likened to the blastoff of a rocket ship. Both substances are described as profound, bewildering, and utterly alien to everyday consciousness, with sought-after spiritual states often going hand in hand with moments of primal fear.

That may be where the similarities end. Unlike DMT, famous for its swirling, intricate geometric patterns and mind-bending alien landscapes, 5-MeO-DMT is not especially visual in nature. Psychedelic aficionados are divided. Some prefer the purity of 5-MeO-DMT, which offers a full spiritual experience without the visual distractions, while others prefer the vibrant, interactive world of DMT and find its 5-MeO variant cold and colorless.

Undoubtedly, it's a substance for serious exploration, not recreation. Many even consider it sacred, as the Yanomami do. Terms such as "oneness," "white light," "pure love," and "ego loss" may sound cribbed from descriptions of religious ecstasy or near-death experiences, but they appear just as often in 5-MeO-DMT narratives. In the moment, users often believe they have died and passed into the afterlife, shedding their human identities as they enter the light. The "ego," or self, simply dissolves, leaving a boundless state of nothingness, completely devoid of the trappings of material life. Lifelong psychedelic researcher Dr. Stan Grof describes it beautifully:

Users often believe they have died and passed into the afterlife, shedding their human identities as they enter the light.

My only reality was a mass of radiant swirling energy of immense proportions that seemed to contain all of existence in a condensed and entirely abstract form. I became Consciousness facing the Absolute. It had the brightness of myriad suns, yet it was not in the same continuum as any light I knew from everyday life. It seemed to be pure consciousness, intelligence, and creative energy transcending all polarities. It was infinite and finite, divine and demonic, terrifying and ecstatic, creative and destructive—all that and much more. I had no concept, no categories for what I was witnessing. I could not maintain a sense of separate existence in the face of such a force. My ordinary identity was shattered and dissolved; I became one with the Source.

Though it can be terrifying, especially when resisted, users who give in to the experience describe it as an oceanic spiritual state—nirvana, infinity, samadhi, or the godhead, depending on whom you ask. One thing they all agree on, though: This state of being defies language. The 5-MeO-DMT void cannot be communicated, analyzed, or comprehended. It can only be experienced.

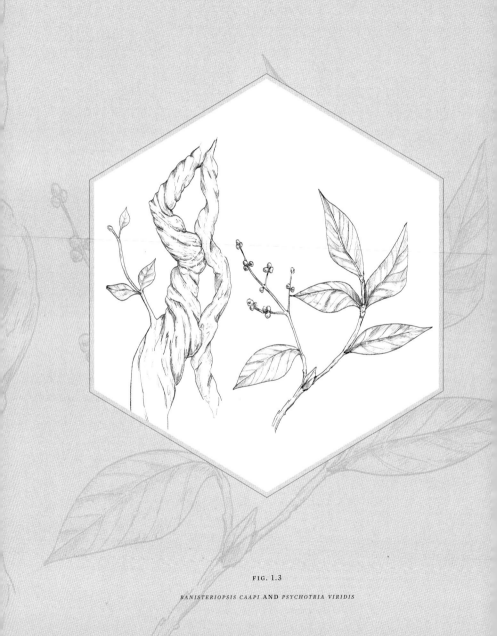

FIG. 1.3

BANISTERIOPSIS CAAPI AND PSYCHOTRIA VIRIDIS

AYAHUASCA

ASSOCIATED WITH *indigeneous tribes of the Amazon rainforest*

ORIGINS AND BACKGROUND

S PIRITUAL MEDICINE OR ESCAPIST DREAM? Toxic hallucinogen or cherished tradition? An intelligent plant spirit with benevolent intentions or a molecular cocktail with an affinity for the brain's receptors? With ayahuasca—derived from a Quechua word meaning, "vine of the spirit," and pronounced *eye-uh-WAHS-kuh*—all the usual arguments about the value of psychedelics are in full force. Some call the bitter drink our species' best shot at salvation, while others dismiss it as an illusory jungle high, more *Fear and Loathing in Peru* than enlightenment in a cup. Few who have tried ayahuasca belong to the latter camp.

The U. S. government maintains that ayahuasca—by virtue of containing DMT, a prohibited substance—is a dangerous drug with no accepted medical use and "a high potential for abuse." Meanwhile, Peru has honored it as a national treasure, recognizing it as "a wise or teaching plant, which shows to initiates the very foundations of the world and its components." There, in the northwestern Amazon rainforest, ayahuasca has been highly revered for many generations.

Most of us are left somewhere in the middle—neither devotee nor cynic. The modern Western mind's approach to this ancient phenomenon is defined, increasingly, by openness and curiosity. This curiosity has boomed in recent years, leading to an explosion of what have been dubbed "spiritual tourists"—those who travel from all over the world to partake in the hallowed ceremonies led by shamans known as *ayahuasqueros*.

Perhaps part of the drink's appeal is, perversely, its unpleasantness—
The New Yorker referred to it as "the drug of choice for the age of kale."
It's an ordeal, not a joyride. For this reason, ayahuasca is rarely encountered
on the black market as a recreational drug.

PREHISTORIC PHARMACISTS AND THE PREPARATION OF AYAHUASCA

Among indigenous tribes in the Amazon, ayahuasca has been a healing medicine
for centuries, if not millennia. To prepare it, they harvest a special selection
of jungle plants and boil them into a concentrated liquid drunk by the cupful.
Though often called a "tea," it isn't your standard cuppa: The resulting sludge
is extremely bitter and takes considerable discipline for most newcomers to
choke down without gagging. Its taste can generously be described as cough
syrup mixed with burnt coffee.

The exact recipe varies, but two ingredients are key: Chacruna is a shrub
whose leaves abound with ayahuasca's main psychoactive ingredient, DMT, the
same molecule vaporized by intrepid consciousness explorers for a brief, intense
trip through alien landscapes (see page 48). Not surprisingly, it's the DMT that
provides ayahuasca with its legendary hallucinatory effects. Occasionally, the
chacruna shrub is replaced by chaliponga, a leafy vine that also contains DMT.

The other main player is *Banisteriopsis caapi*, or simply *caapi*, a woody vine
teeming with chemicals called *harmala alkaloids*. Although it is DMT that
provides the visions, indigenous peoples consider caapi vine to be the tea's most
crucial ingredient. To them, this thick, ropy vine is ayahuasca itself. Shamans
often say the vine provides the journey; the chacruna leaves add the "light" or
visual component. Other common additives include *Brugmansia*, a nightshade
causing delirium and bizarre hallucinations; *Ilex guayusa*, a holly with a high
caffeine content, and tobacco.

Taken by themselves, neither of the two chief ingredients has strong effects.
When ingested, the chacruna's DMT is rapidly metabolized by enzymes before it
ever reaches the brain. That's why, outside the jungle, DMT is most often vaporized

and inhaled; when eaten, it has no effect at all. And the harmala chemicals in the caapi vine, while certainly psychoactive, do not hold a candle to the visionary effects of DMT and other psychedelics.

Taken together, however, the effects are profound. The chemicals in the caapi vine are MAO inhibitors, or MAOIs. They temporarily block the stomach's ability to metabolize DMT, stealthily incapacitating the body's sentries to give DMT free passage into the bloodstream, and, from there, the brain.

How exactly the Amazonian tribes discovered this synergistic combination remains an open question. When asked, shamans simply reply that the plant spirits taught their ancestors which plants to use. In their worldview, ayahuasca is not only a medicine but "La Madre," a maternal entity who shares her wisdom with human beings. As long as man has existed, the spirit of the vine has guided him.

However it came about, this ancient recipe represents an amazing feat: There are at least forty thousand plant species in the Amazon, many of them toxic. Yet, the indigenous people managed to discover the combination of two plants that produces the extraordinary emotional experience known as ayahuasca.

THE EXPERIENCE

In the Amazon, ayahuasca is not considered a drug, but a sacred medicine and spiritual tool. The natives believe each plant has its own spirit, which offers a unique blend of teachings to humanity. The decoction, then, is a sacrament in the truest sense: Composed of benevolent plant intermediaries, it allows partakers to commune directly with the spirit world. Indeed, among many communities, ayahuasca visions represent a higher plane of reality; everyday consciousness is understood to be illusory.

With the guidance of a trusted *curandero*, or healer, native peoples use the vine to purge themselves of evil spirits, connect with their ancestors, and heal various bodily and mental blockages. Aspects that Westerners would normally consider unpleasant side effects, such as vomiting and diarrhea, are regarded by shamans

To shamans, Ayahuasca is not only a medicine but "La Madre," a maternal entity who shares her wisdom with human beings.

as essential characteristics of the experience, a purging of negativity in all its forms. The goal is catharsis, not entertainment.

Ceremonies are conducted in a *maloca*, a communal longhouse made of natural materials, usually round in shape with a thatched roof. For the week before a ceremony, participants are expected to follow a strict diet that includes no red meat, no refined sugar, no alcohol, and no spicy foods; they also abstain from sex.

Participants sit in a circle facing one another, and each is provided a bucket for "purging." The curandero offers each person a cupful of the thick brown tea and the session begins. An ayahuasca ceremony can last from 4 to 8 hours and often consists of two or three cupfuls over the course of the evening.

For the duration of the ceremony—and often throughout the process of mashing and boiling the ingredients beforehand—the shaman sings *icaros*, spiritual songs shamans claim to have learned from the plant spirits themselves. The shaman sings to invoke these spirits and direct the energies flowing in and out of the *maloca*. If someone is having a difficult time with the medicine, the shaman may sing a particular icaro to dispel dark spirits and protect that person from harm. And as any psychedelic user knows, music can be used to intensify or subdue the experience. Against a background of jungle noises that may seem alarming and unfamiliar to nonnatives, the shaman's icaros serve to protect, center, and reassure.

THE RISKS AND REWARDS OF SPIRITUAL TOURISM

Now famous on the world stage, ayahuasca has become a touristic sensation in South America, especially in Peru where it draws thousands of spiritual seekers every year. The intangible, experiential equivalent of Paris's Eiffel Tower or New York's Statue of Liberty, the tea has become recognized not only as a cultural treasure, but also an economic boon to the region.

Iquitos, a city of a half million residents and the largest city in the Peruvian Amazon, has become the unofficial ayahuasca capital of the world. It is also the biggest city anywhere that cannot be reached by road—it is only accessible by air or river. Somewhere between thirty and one hundred ayahuasca centers operate

TWO RICHARDS IN TWO CENTURIES:
HOW THE WEST DISCOVERED AYAHUASCA

Western culture's first recorded encounter with the vine dates to the mid-eighteenth century, when Spanish conquistadors and missionaries reported, "an intoxicating potion ingested for divinatory and other purposes and called *ayahuasca*, which deprives one of his senses and, at times, of his life." These Christian imperialists, whose relationship with indigenous peoples was dictated more by their desire to subdue than to understand, dismissed the medicine as a "diabolical potion."

Later explorers were more open-minded. In the 1850s, the great English botanist Richard Spruce undertook the first scientific study of ayahuasca. As he traveled throughout Peru, Brazil, Venezuela, and Ecuador, he lived among native peoples, learned their languages, and obsessively catalogued local plant species.

In the fourteen years Spruce spent traveling through the Amazon basin and Andes Mountains, he collected some thirty thousand specimens, many of them previously unknown to science. Among them were the first specimens of caapi vine ever studied by white men and seeds of the quinine-rich cinchona tree, whose antimalarial properties had long been recognized by the natives.

The next major explorer to elucidate the mystery of ayahuasca was Richard Evans Schultes. Growing up in Boston, young Richard was fascinated with the Amazon rainforest. At the age of five, his parents read him excerpts of *Notes of a Botanist on the Amazon and Andes*—the diary of none other than Richard Spruce, who became the boy's personal hero. Later, as a biology and botany student at Harvard, Schultes found himself especially drawn to the complex relationships between humans and psychoactive plants and fungi.

Schultes is now considered the father of ethnobotany, the field concerned with the overlap between human cultures and plants. He spent most of the 1940s in the rainforest, armed with little more than an aluminum canoe and a single change of clothes. Like Spruce before him, Schultes collected tens of thousands of specimens, hundreds of them previously undiscovered. At least 120 species have been named for him.

In 1953, Schultes returned to the United States and became a professor at his alma mater. His was one of the first voices to draw attention to the alarming rate of destruction of the Amazon rainforest and with it, the knowledge and cultures of mestizo peoples. A prolific author, one of his most enduring works is *Plants of the Gods*, a book he coauthored with Albert Hofmann, the discoverer of LSD.

Schultes observed firsthand the central importance of ayahuasca in these people's way of life and drank the tea on many occasions. He demonstrated the presence of DMT-containing chacruna and chaliponga leaves in ayahuasca preparations and thus set the stage for a deeper understanding of the jungle elixir.

For someone whose life's work would prove so influential to psychedelic enthusiasts, Schultes was remarkably sober and grounded. He thought little of his Harvard colleague, the psychedelic icon Timothy Leary, remarking that Leary understood so little about biology that he misspelled the Latin names of hallucinogenic plants. In a famous exchange with William S. Burroughs, Schultes replied succinctly to the writer's description of an intense, transcendent ayahuasca experience: "That's funny, Bill, all I saw was colors."

in and around Iquitos, plus many disreputable operators offering the drink to make a quick buck from unwitting foreigners.

These would-be shamans are a real problem: Though the boom in spiritual tourism has brought money and interest to the region, it has also provided ample opportunity for shady characters to pass themselves off as skilled shamans. Some are simply careless and inexperienced, not yet ready to manage the intense emotions of a group of rookie gringos who may be tasting the vine for the first time. Others are manipulative con men and predators: There have been multiple cases of women sexually assaulted by their so-called shamans. Perpetrated by men posing as trusted guides in a sacred therapeutic process, these crimes represent an especially vicious betrayal of trust.

Although ayahuasca can cause complications for those on certain medications or with a history of mental illness, it is very rare for death to result from consuming the drink alone. In 2012, an eighteen-year-old American died in mysterious circumstances after consuming a high dose of ayahuasca at a healing center. The shaman, concerned for his center's reputation, buried the man in a field and lied to police and the boy's family before eventually coming clean.

Two years later, a young English man suffered a fatal reaction to the brew in Colombia, and his body was left roadside by the locals. In 2015, a Canadian man stabbed another man in self-defense when the latter, under the influence of ayahuasca, became violent and attacked him.

Shocking stories like these make for sensational headlines, but they are the exception, not the rule. Still, the risks are real. Travelers are warned to conduct extensive research and tread with extreme caution when considering an ayahuasca session in an unfamiliar country.

BEYOND THE JUNGLE

Like the double helix formed by caapi vine as it twines around itself in the jungle, ayahuasca and the modern world have joined in an intimate embrace. The exchange goes both ways: As thousands of pilgrims flock to the Amazon in search of healing and wholeness, Madre Ayahuasca sows her seeds in the urban centers of the world. For people in cities such as San Francisco, New York, and London, where underground sessions have become a regular occurrence, it's no longer necessary to book a flight to Iquitos to take the sacrament.

Urban *curanderos* model their healing circles after traditional ceremonies, but of course it's not quite the same—Westerners, no matter how well intentioned, have a host of different biases and assumptions than indigenous peoples in the Amazon rainforest. Ceremonies have become popular both in informal settings and as sacred rituals within syncretic neo-Christian churches such as Santo Daime and the União do Vegetal.

These two churches are especially interesting because of their legal status in the United States. Much like the Native American Church, whose religious use of peyote is protected by law, members of Santo Daime and União do Vegetal are exempt from the federal ban on DMT.

In the Santo Daime tradition, which combines core Christian beliefs with elements of African animism and South American shamanistic practices, parishioners take part in a highly ritualized drinking of the brew, which they call *Daime*. Each ceremony consists of prayer, dancing, singing, and communing with healing energies via the sacrament.

Santo Daime found a champion in their home country of Brazil, whose drug agency undertook a seven-year study on the effects of ayahuasca before concluding that the tea did not have adverse effects on its users. "To the contrary," wrote the judgment, "it appears to orient them toward seeking social contentment in an orderly and productive way." Thanks to this landmark decision, ayahuasca has been exempted from Brazilian controlled substance regulation since 1992.

União do Vegetal (UDV), Portuguese for "union of the plants," was founded by a Brazilian rubber tapper in 1961. Like Santo Daime, UDV's sacrament follows the traditional ayahuasca recipe of caapi vine and chacruna leaves, though it calls the medicine by its Portuguese name, *Hoasca*. Hoasca sessions last about 4 hours and emphasize "the enhancement of mental concentration and solemn reflection on the teachings of our guide, Mestre Gabriel, and Jesus."

It's no longer necessary to book a flight to Iquitos to take the sacrament.

In the United States, a series of court decisions in 2006 and 2009 found in favor of the UDV and Santo Daime churches, protecting their use of ayahuasca as legitimate religious activities. However, the protection only applies to these two organizations. For all others, ayahuasca remains a Schedule I substance with stiff penalties for possession and sale.

HEALING PROPERTIES

Proponents claim that a dose of ayahuasca lowers their defenses, allowing them to unravel their traumas and deep-rooted insecurities with uncommon clarity. Although an abundance of anecdotal evidence suggests beneficial effects on a variety of mental conditions, very little clinical research has been conducted. Early results are limited but promising.

A 2007 study of long-term members of the Santo Daime religion showed that participants experienced reduced anxiety, panic, and hopelessness in the short term. Two years later, researchers found that beginners who drank the brew regularly over six months scored higher on surveys of emotional functioning.

Of greater interest are ayahuasca's long-term effects. Advocates claim it helps people overcome trauma, anxiety, depression, and addiction to drugs including alcohol and tobacco. But where's the science?

A landmark 1996 study led by Dr. Charles Grob, a luminary in the field of psychedelic science, examined a small group of UDV members who had consumed Hoasca regularly for at least ten years. He found that although most of the experimental subjects had previously suffered from mental and behavioral problems, including alcoholism, depression, and anxiety, none met the criteria for any disorder at the time of the study.

Both the unusually high incidence of prior mental illnesses and their apparent resolution are enlightening: On one hand, as something of an entheogenic self-help community, Santo Daime tends to attract troubled and suffering people. On the other hand, their recovery coincides with their membership in the church

These results are preliminary, but promising.

and regular attendance of "works," though it's impossible to establish causation in a study of such limited scope.

A 2008 study of American Santo Daime members found similar results. Of the thirty-two people interviewed, twenty-four had a history of substance addiction, and nineteen had previously met criteria for psychiatric conditions that ranged from bulimia and phobias to depression and post-traumatic stress disorder. At the time of the study, the vast majority of these issues remained in remission— a remarkable feat the participants attributed to their church membership and weekly Daime sessions.

In a Canadian study in 2013, twelve people struggling with substance addictions were given ayahuasca along with group counseling sessions over four days. Six months later, the subjects reported a decrease in their problematic drug use and improved measures of hopefulness, empowerment, and mindfulness. All indicated they experienced lasting positive effects from the retreat.

These results are preliminary, but promising. The medical world watches eagerly to see if science will continue to vindicate the healing power of the ancient jungle potion.

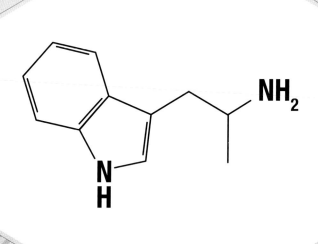

FIG. 1.4

N,N-DIMETHYLTRYPTAMINE

DISCOVERED

Used since antiquity;
synthesized in 1931;
discovered in plants in 1946;
discovered in humans in 1972

DURATION

15 minutes when vaporized

DMT

ASSOCIATED WITH *author and speaker Terence McKenna and psychiatrist and researcher Dr. Rick Strassman*

ORIGINS AND BACKGROUND

THOUGH OFTEN OVERSHADOWED BY MORE POPULAR COMPOUNDS such as LSD and psilocybin, DMT is in many ways the quintessential psychedelic. Unlike its better-known chemical cousins, DMT, short for *N,N*-dimethyltryptamine, occurs naturally in a wide variety of plants and animals, including the human body. Although it is by far the most common psychedelic in nature, DMT rarely occurs in concentrations high enough to cause intoxication. Its purpose in humans and other organisms remains a mystery, but its apparent ubiquity in nature seems to indicate a fundamental role—if not as a neurotransmitter, then at least as a chemical building block for other important compounds.

For many centuries, DMT has featured as one of two chief ingredients in ayahuasca, the plant-based sacrament revered by Amazonian tribes. More recently, this once-obscure brew has attracted waves of "spiritual tourists" to the jungle in search of healing, cleansing, and catharsis. DMT's role in this traditional context is covered in the separate ayahuasca chapter of this book (see page 35). This chapter focuses on the isolated compound, which in the twentieth century has emerged as an entheogen and exploratory tool in its own right.

Though the substance is not, gram for gram, especially potent—an effective dose requires one hundred times more material than LSD—a full DMT "breakthrough" is widely considered by seasoned explorers of consciousness as one of the most powerful of all visionary experiences.

Although all of us produce and metabolize trace amounts of DMT every day, higher doses are definitely not for the fainthearted. A peerless, sublime, and extremely fast-paced entheogen, DMT commands respect from even the most fearless explorers of inner space.

BEYOND AYAHUASCA

Extracted DMT comes in powder or crystal form and ranges in color from white to yellow. It has a light but distinctive fragrance, reminiscent of sweet flowers, but when vaporized, takes on a pungent odor somewhat like burning plastic. DMT is occasionally injected, although this requires specialized materials and skills. The pure compound can be consumed orally, as with ayahuasca, but must be combined with another chemical to prevent stomach enzymes from breaking down the DMT. Such pharmaceutical analogs of the jungle brew are known, fittingly enough, as "pharmahuasca."

Most often, DMT is vaporized in a glass pipe and inhaled. This has the twofold result of compressing the timeframe of the experience while greatly intensifying its effects. An oral formulation such as ayahuasca lasts between 3 and 5 hours; vaporized DMT is closer to 15 minutes.

A newer formulation has gained popularity in recent years. Changa, a smoking blend of DMT-infused plant materials, originated in Australia in the early 2000s and has since found favor among DMT enthusiasts around the world. Like ayahuasca, changa blends usually feature both DMT and other compounds, called MAOIs, which potentiate DMT's effects. Changa may also feature nonpsychoactive herbs, such as peppermint, lavender, and blue lotus. In duration and intensity, changa lies somewhere between vaporized DMT and traditional ayahuasca. Its many advocates appreciate the slower onset, longer duration, and altogether more manageable experience when compared to vaporizing pure DMT.

DMT IN THE 1950S AND '60S

Although it played a central role in shamanic ceremonies in the Amazon for many centuries, the compound DMT was only synthesized by Western scientists in 1931 and not discovered in plant sources until 1946. Even then, researchers did not know they had uncovered a powerful psychedelic.

The first insight into DMT's astonishing psychoactive effects came in 1956 from a Hungarian psychiatrist and chemist named Stephen Szára. A true explorer and experimentalist, Szára consumed larger and larger oral doses of DMT, all to no effect. Correctly supposing that the gut might be metabolizing the compound before it could reach the brain, Szára decided to try an alternative route. When he injected himself with DMT, he discovered the effects were consistent with descriptions of LSD and mescaline, but much shorter in duration. His description represents the first ever report of injected DMT.

> *The hallucinations consisted of moving, brilliantly colored Oriental motifs, and later I saw wonderful scenes altering very rapidly. The faces of the people seemed to be masks. My emotional state was elevated sometimes up to euphoria . . . My consciousness was completely filled by hallucinations, and my attention was firmly bound to them . . .*

Word soon got out to adventurous psychedelic circles. The Beat novelist William S. Burroughs became one of the first to try this mysterious new chemical. It was not to his liking. In a letter to Timothy Leary, Burroughs explained that his DMT experience was, "completely and horribly real and involved unendurable pain."

In the early 1960s, just as he was ramping up the Harvard Psilocybin Project, Leary began hearing whisperings of this powerful new psychedelic. Though Burroughs had warned him of its terrifying nature, Leary's curiosity got the best of him. Although it never found its way into his psychedelic research program at Harvard, injected DMT would later become a mainstay in Millbrook, Leary's psychedelic haven in upstate New York.

DMT commands respect from even the most fearless explorers of inner space.

In his book *High Priest,* Leary described his first-ever DMT experience in the company of a few close friends:

> *The people present were transfigured . . . godlike creatures . . . we were all united as one organism. Beneath the radiant surface I could see the delicate, wondrous body machinery of each person, the network of muscle and vein and bone— exquisitely beautiful and all joined, all part of the same process.*

At that time, DMT wasn't for the squeamish—the stigma of injecting drugs kept all but the most dedicated explorers from trying the new psychedelic. But it wasn't long before Nick Sand, one of the two clandestine chemists responsible for the iconic Orange Sunshine acid of the 1960s, made a groundbreaking discovery: Freebase DMT could be smoked.

Vaporizing changed the nature of the experience tremendously, from a 1-hour ride to a 10-minute rocket ship through hyperspace. This marked the beginning of DMT's reputation as "the businessman's trip," a chemical of incredible power that blasted the user to another dimension and back in a matter of minutes.

Though it never gained widespread recognition as a 1960s countercultural icon the way cannabis and LSD did, DMT commanded respect as a powerful substance among those in the know—and has continued to amass a dedicated following since its discovery.

THE EXPERIENCE

When vaporized, DMT's effects are indescribably intense and nearly immediate. Users speak of attempting to inhale a second or third hit while the room dissolves into fractals around them. A euphoric, tingling "buzz" traverses the user's body, often coinciding with auditory hallucinations such as a rising tone or sounds that resemble crinkling plastic. There is a strong impression of being launched into an alien dimension. Indeed, the onset is so rapid that many users refer to it as "blastoff."

According to Terence McKenna, within a minute of vaporizing DMT you enter into "the Dome"—a space "crawling with geometric hallucinations, very brightly colored, very iridescent with deep sheens and very high, reflective surfaces—everything is machinelike and polished and throbbing with energy." This bewildering phantasmagoria keeps shifting at a blistering pace, and some users complain it's too fast to be of any shamanic or therapeutic use.

DMT HYPERSPACE

A consciousness explorer, author, and prolific speaker, Terence McKenna was, more than anything else, a supreme storyteller. A popular lecturer on the psychedelic circuit throughout the 1990s, McKenna riffed on psychedelics, alien beings, and any other topic that captured his expansive curiosity.

McKenna first tried DMT as a student at Berkeley in 1965 and was astonished at the kaleidoscopic worlds he discovered within. He later credited that initial taste with jumpstarting his "commitment to the psychedelic experience"—an endeavor that would occupy him for the rest of his life.

Throughout the 1980s and '90s, with "Just Say No" antidrug propaganda in full swing, McKenna's remained one of the clearest and loudest voices advocating the use of psychedelics as self-exploratory tools. An iconoclast and fearless critic of society, McKenna called for people to take psychedelics to see through the "cultural programming" that obstructed their minds. Psychedelics, he said, "open you up to the possibility that everything you know is wrong." In some ways, he was the Timothy Leary of the rave generation, though certainly polarizing and less messianic than his predecessor.

Although he died in 2000 of brain cancer, McKenna's immense influence on psychedelic culture continues today. Recordings of his lectures, featuring outlandish descriptions of DMT "hyperspace," incisive social commentary, and fringe theories of human evolution and alien contact have amassed millions of views online.

McKenna's erudite, even poetic descriptions of what he called the "un-Englishable" experience of DMT consciousness—delivered with wry wit and his distinctive nasal voice—have been instrumental to the substance's surge in popularity over the last two decades. The experience, he said, is "of a fundamentally different order than any other experience this side of the yawning grave."

By all accounts, DMT is an intensely visual experience. But it's more than just a kaleidoscopic roller coaster—for many people, it offers a truly spiritual connection. Nick Sand described it as, "the doorway to the intensely personal temple of our own sacredness." He said:

DMT creates a wellspring into a type of infinite space. You can feel and taste it, as it moves through your whole being like a cool refreshing breeze on a hot sticky day. Like a mother's soothing touch on your fevered brow, but much deeper and more profound. You can feel the wind of the Divine blowing through your soul.

DR. RICK STRASSMAN AND PSYCHEDELIC RESEARCH

With the passage of the Controlled Substances Act in 1970, DMT became illegal, along with mescaline, psilocybin, and many other substances. Among those committed to obtaining DMT, this prohibition has had little effect—homebrew explorers can easily extract it from a variety of legal plant sources. But it did stop scientific research. Stephen Szára, who had emigrated from Hungary to the United States and continued studying DMT under the auspices of the National Institutes of Health, was forced to halt this fascinating avenue of research. So was Szára's colleague, Nobel Prize winner Julius Axelrod, who in 1972 published the first study demonstrating the presence of DMT in healthy human brain tissue—a study that paved the way for the modern understanding of DMT as pervasive in nature and, perhaps, fundamental to the healthy functioning of all plants and animals.

Though technically legal to research, the new prohibition had enacted such a complex system of approvals that for the next twenty years, even the most dedicated consciousness scientists turned their attention to other matters.

One scientist, however, was not deterred. After a laborious two-year process to secure the necessary permissions, Dr. Rick Strassman, a psychiatrist at the University of New Mexico, began the first major study of psychedelics in human subjects in decades. From 1990 to 1995, Strassman injected sixty volunteers with around four hundred doses of DMT and interviewed them about their experiences. He documented the results in his book *DMT: The Spirit Molecule*—a term he coined to reflect the many similarities between DMT trips and religious experiences.

The results were fascinating. Volunteers frequently reported they left their bodies and entered an exotic, nonphysical realm. Many people felt they were dying—but by surrendering to the experience, many were able to transform this into a positive and cathartic event. Some volunteers experienced DMT as a sort of accelerated psychotherapy that helped them confront and resolve unconscious anxieties. Many experienced what Strassman described as a transpersonal or mystical state, consisting of feelings of oneness, connection, and rebirth, often with profound spiritual connotations.

MACHINE ELVES, SPIRITS, AND ENTITIES

One of the strangest and most hotly debated aspects of the DMT experience is the appearance of otherworldly entities—organic, shapeshifting forms of pure energy who communicate telepathically and give the unmistakable impression of independent intelligence. It sounds outrageous, yet reports of such "DMT entities" are surprisingly common. And yet with other psychedelics, such encounters are very rare—it seems DMT alone provides access to the inhabited regions of the far shores of consciousness.

For Strassman, the appearance of these beings proved to be one of the most intriguing and unexpected aspects of his study. More than half of all volunteers encountered "'entities,' 'beings,' 'aliens,' 'guides,' and 'helpers'," which took the forms of "clowns, reptiles, mantises, bees, spiders, cacti, and stick figures." Although many encounters were benign, some volunteers perceived them as "ornery," "prankish," and even "sinister." One described the experience as, "like being possessed," and other reports had frightening undertones of alien abductions. Perhaps most shocking of all, many volunteers believed these entities were completely real, long after the effects of the drug wore off.

Terence McKenna described these hyperdimensional creatures as, "jeweled self-dribbling basketballs," "chirping fractal denizens of the unconscious," and—most famously—"mercurial and mischievous machine elves . . . strange teachers whose marvelous singing makes intricate toys out of the air and out of their own continually tranforming body geometries."

Though "machine elves" has become an indelible part of the modern DMT lexicon, McKenna was hardly the first to encounter foreign beings while under the influence of DMT. Indeed, Amazonian natives have been communing with spirits for thousands of years by taking ayahuasca. And as early as 1958, Szára described one of his research subjects encountering "strange creatures, dwarves or something."

These entities have been variously interpreted as aliens, spirits, angels, emissaries from a parallel dimension, or even long-dead ancestors. Others dismiss them as exceptionally convincing hallucinations, like characters in a dream.

Nick Sand—the chemist who discovered that DMT could be vaporized, and a man with thousands of trips under his belt—came to this conclusion:

> *The beings and creatures I've seen have been curious and various, but they have never looked like anyone I've ever seen, nor any mythical creature from history. . . . Although they were totally original and amazing, never did I feel that they were strangers. I recognized them immediately. They had a bizarre but faintly and curiously familiar feeling to them. I think that this is significant, in that the lesson is one of personal responsibility. These are our creatures created by the infinitely capable creative force to teach us about ourselves. They are mirrors that help us do the difficult job of looking at ourselves, and remembering who we are.*

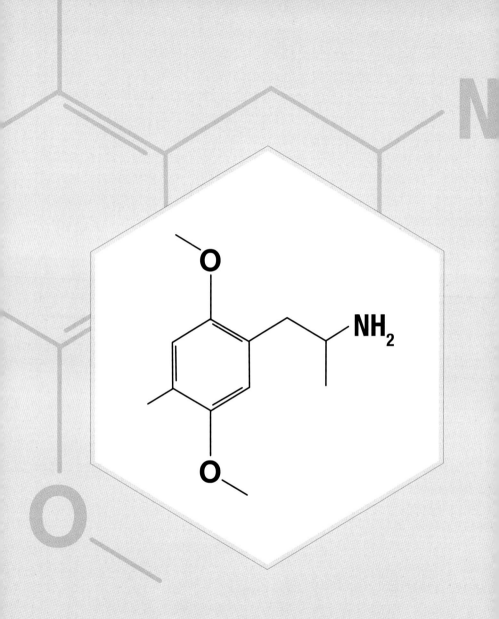

FIG. 1.5

2,5-DIMETHOXY-4-METHYLAMPHETAMINE

DOM AND THE DOx FAMILY

ALSO KNOWN AS STP

ORIGINS AND BACKGROUND

THE BEST KNOWN OF ALL THE PSYCHEDELIC AMPHETAMINES, the DOx family is famous for being both incredibly potent and long-lived. Though undeniably psychedelic, the DOx experience is more endurance race than sprint: slow out of the gate, long and intense in the middle, and taking 24 hours or more to finish. Trailing stimulation and other aftereffects can linger for several days. Consisting of DOM and dozens of other chemicals, such as DOI—and likely many more yet to be unearthed— the DOx series has been delighting, terrifying, and trying the patience of hippies and psychonauts since the first compound was discovered in 1963.

Alexander Shulgin discovered the DOx series by modifying one chemical skeleton in many different ways. The "x" in DOx is just a placeholder: Attach a bromine and you get DOB; iodine, DOI; and chlorine, DOC. Add a methyl group, and you get the granddaddy of them all, DOM—the first that Shulgin discovered and, thanks to ill-fated experimentation by hippies on the West Coast, the first to attract attention from law enforcement, the media, and the medical community.

Shulgin first created DOM in 1963 while researching psychedelics for the Dow Chemical company. He and his friends found 3 to 5 milligrams produced strong effects. Many users report a pleasant "body high" that amplifies every tactile sensation into a wave of pleasure, along with heightened vision and hearing. Elaborate hallucinations are common, and users may find themselves immersed in fully realized fantasies, especially with their eyes closed. After only 5 milligrams, one of Shulgin's guinea pigs wrote, "I knew what it was like to look across the brink to insanity." At 10 milligrams, Shulgin reported, "DOM has the glory and the doom sealed up in it." And 12 milligrams produced tremors that felt "like poisoning."

Imagine the madness when DOM first hit the streets of San Francisco in the form of 20-milligram tablets. Distributed as STP, no one at the time knew the substance was, in fact, DOM. Said to stand for "serenity, tranquility, peace," STP sowed only havoc and confusion among the Haight-Ashbury hippies who took it. Chemists quickly halved the dose, but 10 milligrams still guaranteed an intense 24-hour affair.

Thousands of such doses were distributed to attendees of the Human Be-In, an event held in Golden Gate Park in 1967, a few months before the Summer of Love. Because LSD had been banned in California the year before, the time was ripe for a fresh alternative to take center stage.

But DOM's debut was an unmitigated disaster. The high dose was compounded by DOM's unusually slow onset—many people, feeling no effects after 1 hour, took another tablet, or even two. This proved to be a huge mistake. As the Beat poet Allen Ginsberg chanted mantras, the Grateful Dead played a heady set, and Timothy Leary urged everyone to "Turn on, tune in, drop out," thousands of people began to freak out.

Bay Area hospitals were soon flooded with tripping hippies. Time proved to be the best medicine—eventually all users returned to terra firma, though probably more than a few swore off psychedelics for life. Thankfully, nobody died. The main casualty was DOM, whose reputation soured overnight.

In hindsight, the condemnation was premature. Far from revealing any poisonous properties of DOM, the Human Be-In mishap vividly demonstrated the need for regulation and education concerning recreational drugs. If it weren't for the spinning wheels of Prohibition, spurring users to ever newer and more obscure substances, the hippies probably would have taken good old LSD that day— a familiar trip with very low toxicity and a more manageable timeline of effects.

RAM DASS AND KEN KESEY ON "STP"

Several 1960s luminaries have testified to DOM's extraordinary effects. Dr. Richard Alpert, the professor who started the Harvard Psilocybin Project with Timothy Leary and is now better known as the guru Ram Dass, first tried the compound in a Manhattan apartment. After an overly intense experience culminating in an attempt to walk out of a high-rise window, he disavowed the substance.

Upon trying it again, after five days of fasting in the Taos valley of New Mexico, Alpert described it as, "an extraordinary, extraordinary trip. I was *really* impressed. I still thought it was maybe too strong an agent for most people . . . But it was certainly a profound psychedelic experience."

Ken Kesey, the author and psychedelic icon who led a bus full of his Merry Pranksters on an acid-fueled cross-country journey, was less enthusiastic. After taking way too much DOM, he and his friends found themselves subjected to a "readjusting" at the hands of a sinister alien presence.

"We didn't hold it together," Kesey explained. "And I forgot something . . . I lost a thing we take for granted, something that's been forged over I don't know how many thousands of years of human effort, and it's now in us." He compared it to navigating a boat adrift. "When I reached for the tiller behind me, after the

STP, I found that it wasn't there anymore. I no longer knew what man was doing cruising along through the world."

That's pretty bleak stuff. But perhaps, as with the debacle in San Francisco, Kesey's existential crisis boiled down to a matter of dosage. According to him, Grateful Dead soundman and clandestine chemist Owsley Stanley, "was taking the stuff out with a spoon and letting people snort or lick it off."

If there's a lesson to be learned from the excesses of DOM in the 1960s, surely it comes down to this: Know your substance, and know your dose. Going overboard with any psychedelic is a good way to wind up in the hospital— or lost at sea, grasping for the tiller that makes us human.

DOI'S CONTRIBUTION TO SCIENCE

In the DOx family, DOI is most noteworthy for its considerable contribution to science. Hundreds of published papers have utilized the chemical in some way. The iodine atom in DOI can be replaced with a radioactive isotope, which makes it very useful when combined with an imaging technique called *positron emission tomography*, or PET. As the DOI binds to serotonin receptors throughout the body, the radioactive atom acts as a sort of beacon, allowing researchers to peer into the molecular pathways of the body like never before.

One pioneering study showed that DOI reduces inner-eye pressure, which could prove useful in treating glaucoma. Another team found that it suppresses—with remarkable potency—a natural protein that induces inflammation. DOI could lead to completely new treatments for degenerative diseases such as Alzheimer's and rheumatoid arthritis, in which chronic inflammation plays a key role.

DOI also appears to be effective in preventing asthma—at least in mice. Most serotonin-triggering psychedelics have captured medical interest for their mental effects, but in fact, serotonin and its receptors are found all over the body, including the lungs. In a 2015 study, mice exposed to an allergic stimulus reacted in a way similar to asthma. But when they were administered airborne DOI prior to receiving the stimulus, the mice continued breathing normally—the asthma disappeared. It would take some time to develop DOI into a medicine for humans, but these findings open the door to an altogether new mode of asthma treatment.

There are a whole host of DOx compounds, many of them yet untested. Shulgin's brilliance lay not only in mapping new molecular territories and pushing the frontiers of consciousness forward but in providing tantalizing leads for future explorers. Shulgin was convinced that still more variants of his DOx creations would prove psychoactive and extended an open invitation to the chemical trailblazers of the future.

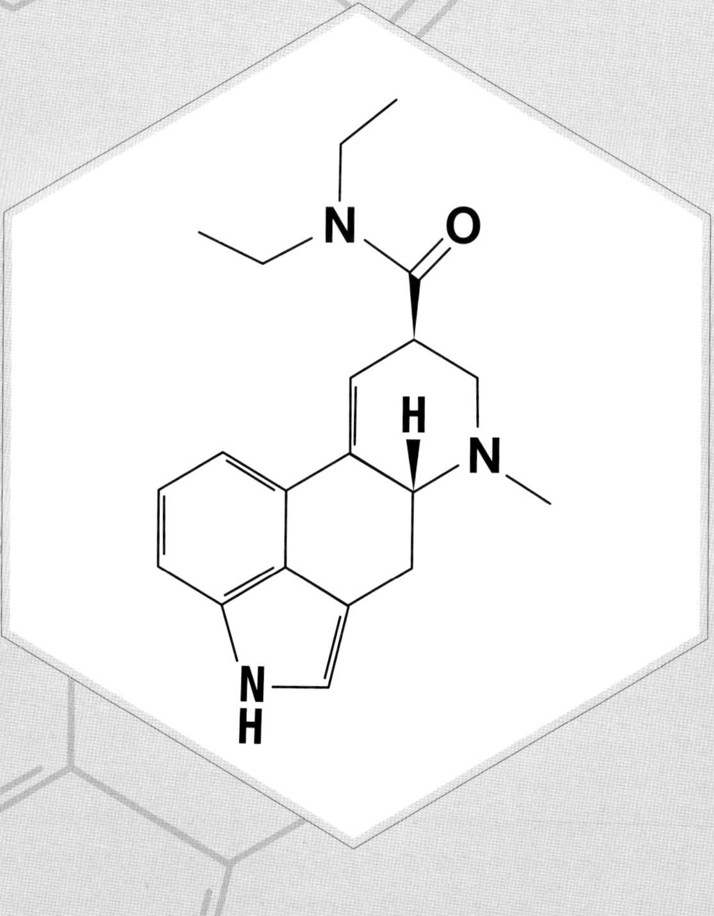

FIG. 1.6

LYSERGIC ACID DIETHYLAMIDE

DISCOVERED

Synthesized in 1938;
psychedelic properties
discovered in 1943 by Swiss
chemist Albert Hofmann

LSD

DURATION

8 to 12 hours

ASSOCIATED WITH *1960s counterculture, the Beatles, the Grateful Dead, Timothy Leary, Ken Kesey*

ORIGINS AND BACKGROUND

ALTHOUGH IT'S THE MOST FAMOUS AND WELL RESEARCHED of all psychedelics, LSD is also, in the long view, one of humanity's newest. Discovered serendipitously by a Swiss chemist in 1938, LSD has since emerged as a countercultural icon, therapeutic medicine, military brainwashing tool, and even a religious sacrament. For many, it defines the term "psychedelic," bringing to mind the 1960s heyday where rock bands, artists, writers, and seekers of all stripes became heavily influenced by this new and earth-shattering substance.

Some substances, upon their discovery, are developed into medicines; others become addictive vices; and still others fade into obscurity. LSD carved its own path, defying all expectations and weaving itself into the tapestry of history. Also known as acid, it became so tightly bound to the zeitgeist of the 1960s that its association with that era still echoes in the collective memory.

LSD's fame was also its undoing. Any substance that becomes popular among countercultural figures risks drawing the ire of the authorities. Although it had been prescribed to tens of thousands of people in the 1950s and studied as a therapeutic treatment for everything from alcoholism to depression, LSD was outlawed in 1968. Yet, it soldiered on as an underground substance and is enjoying a recent resurgence of scientific research.

LSD was, perhaps, the preeminent mind-altering substance of the twentieth century, and, even today, is the standard by which all other psychedelics are judged.

FORMS AND METHODS

Pure LSD is a white crystalline powder with no odor. Because of its incredible potency, however, most users never encounter the pure compound. Most frequently it is dissolved onto "blotter paper"—absorbent paper that is perforated to allow easy removal of individual square doses and often decorated with outlandish designs. Occasionally, LSD comes as a liquid solution, kept in something like an eyedropper that allows easy and consistent dosing.

An active dose is so tiny as to be invisible, and a very large dose would appear no bigger than a grain of sand. LSD's exceptional potency surpasses that of psilocybin, DMT, and mescaline by several orders of magnitude. Like most other classical psychedelics, LSD appears to exert its effects by interacting with the brain's serotonin system.

LSD is also a fragile molecule, breaking down when exposed to light, heat, or air. Usually, LSD is simply eaten or left on the tongue and absorbed via the gums. Today, a number of obscure synthetic chemicals are frequently passed off as genuine LSD. This has led to a prudent saying among recreational users: "If it's bitter, it's a spitter." As LSD has no flavor and most research chemicals are distinctly bitter, the taste serves as an imperfect but somewhat reliable indicator of a dose's quality.

A FORTUITOUS DISCOVERY

LSD owes its existence to a Swiss chemist named Albert Hofmann. While employed by Sandoz, a pharmaceutical company based in Basel, Switzerland, Hofmann was investigating derivatives of ergot, a parasitic fungus that contaminates rye grains and has been responsible for a number of deadly outbreaks of food poisoning throughout history. As it often happens, this natural poison turned out to offer some medical benefits. In 1938, Hofmann synthesized the twenty-fifth derivative of lysergic acid— an ergot-based molecule—and named it LSD-25. After limited testing with animals, it was deemed unremarkable and shelved.

But five years later, motivated by what he called "a peculiar presentiment," Hofmann decided to resynthesize the chemical. In a fortuitous error, he accidentally ingested a tiny amount. Though less than a full-on psychedelic trip, the effects commanded the chemist's attention. Hofmann began feeling restless and dizzy. Lying down, he found himself in a "not unpleasant intoxicatedlike state, characterized by an extremely stimulated imagination." The chemist could only watch as his mind's eye was bombarded with an "uninterrupted stream of fantastic pictures, extraordinary shapes with intense, kaleidoscopic play of colors."

BICYCLE DAY

Hofmann was intrigued. Three days later, he embarked on a second voyage—this time on purpose. To be safe, he measured a conservative amount: 250 micrograms, a mere quarter of a milligram, surely too little to produce any serious effects. He wasn't counting on his new discovery being among the most potent psychoactive compounds known to humankind.

In his lab notebook, he managed to write three terse lines before drifting off, overcome by "dizziness, feelings of anxiety, visual distortions, symptoms of paralysis, [and the] desire to laugh." Alarmed, he asked his lab assistant to escort him home. Due to wartime restrictions on automobile usage, they were forced to take bicycles. It's a strange and memorable image: Amid the carnage of World War II, two chemists bicycle through Basel, one of them serving as LSD's first guinea pig, looking a bit perplexed as he maneuvers through once-familiar streets.

He couldn't have known it then, but this chemical experiment would mark the beginning of a new era of human consciousness. Hofmann's discovery represented a psychedelic "first contact," the very first interface between the human mind and a novel molecule that would change history. Today, Bicycle Day is celebrated every April 19 by LSD enthusiasts around the world, commemorating that momentous bike ride.

LSD's exceptional potency surpasses that of psilocybin, DMT, and mescaline by several orders of magnitude.

The trip did not start on a pleasant note, however. Hofmann found himself besieged by "threatening forms," and everything he saw "wavered and was distorted as if seen in a curved mirror."

Safe at home, on his sofa, he did not fare any better.

> *Every exertion of my will, every attempt to put an end to the disintegration of the outer world and the dissolution of my ego, seemed to be wasted effort. . . . I was seized by the dreadful fear of going insane. I was taken to another world, another place, another time. . . . Was I dying? Was this the transition?*

The chemist became the first LSD subject to mistake the experience of "ego death" for the more permanent kind, but he would not be the last.

As time wore on, though, his fears began to dissipate. The family doctor arrived and assured Hofmann he was the very picture of health—the only abnormal symptom appeared to be extremely dilated pupils.

Eventually, Hofmann discovered he was able to enjoy his unusual state of mind. The "fantastic images," he later wrote, were

> *. . . exploding in colored fountains, rearranging and hybridizing themselves in constant flux. It was particularly remarkable how every acoustic perception, such as the sound of a door handle or a passing automobile, became transformed into optical perceptions. Every sound generated a vividly changing image, with its own consistent form and color.*

The chemist knew right away he'd discovered something special. Between its incredible potency, its apparent safety, and especially its ability to produce profound shifts in consciousness, he expected LSD would have a bright future in psychiatry. What he didn't count on was anyone wanting to take it recreationally—surely the experience's intensity would dissuade any casual users.

Those who've had the honor of dissolving into these boundless depths often rank it as the pinnacle of life itself.

LSD takes 40 to 90 minutes to kick in; once it does, there's no backing out. The full experience lasts from 8 to 12 hours.

In a full-blown acid trip, there is often a sense of openness, childlike wonder, and a heightened emotional sensitivity that can lead to indescribable bliss and contentment or to anxiety, paranoia, and abject terror. Colors become more vivid, borders bleed into each other, and people's facial expressions become impossibly poignant, hilarious, and grotesque by turns. Swirling patterns swim across every surface, taking the form of infinite fractals, elaborate geometric structures, or even recognizable faces. Cognitive shifts lead to nonlinear thought patterns, compassionate yet honest self-analysis, a renegotiation of old assumptions and habits, expansive curiosity, and, in some cases, fears about going insane or dying.

Trips vary tremendously based on many circumstances. Seemingly minor thoughts or environmental cues can send a naïve user flying into a sublime state of oneness or spiraling into a hellish spiritual crisis. As Albert Hofmann's maiden voyage demonstrates, the two extremes may even occur in the same trip.

One of the hallmarks of a deep acid experience is the dissolution of what is commonly known as the ego—the self, the "I," the conscious being with its own experiences and memories, distinct from the rest of the universe. This "ego death" can be terrifying. But if the user surrenders to it, it can also be beautiful—a sense of oneness, of absolutely boundless and infinite love, a state indistinguishable from spontaneous religious experiences described by monks, prophets, and ascetics since time immemorial. For committed psychonauts, ego death is the holy grail of tripping. Those who've had the honor of dissolving into these boundless depths often rank it as the pinnacle of life itself.

THE 1940S AND '50S

After Hofmann's discovery, Sandoz began marketing LSD under the name Delysid as a therapeutic agent in the mid-1940s. It was also considered an excellent tool for producing a "model psychosis," and many psychiatrists sampled it with the aim of better understanding their patients' schizophrenia. The press was very positive, and LSD was regarded as the wunderkind of psychiatry, with broad applications and exotic, if intimidating, effects.

In the 1950s, its profile in science and the media continued to grow. Over a thousand new studies were published, demonstrating the compound's apparent benefits in treating everything from neurosis and depression to autism and—paradoxically, given the prevailing view that LSD induced temporary psychosis—schizophrenia. The results were frequently positive but marred by what, today, would be considered poor methodology; specifically, they lacked the double-blind, placebo-controlled methods that are the hallmarks of modern psychology.

One lasting advancement was in neurochemistry, where LSD studies proved instrumental in clarifying the role of serotonin in the brain. Serotonin, scientists learned, is a fundamental chemical messenger that affects mood, appetite, learning, memory, and sleep. Almost all classical psychedelics are now thought to act primarily through serotonin receptors.

Many of the early LSD studies focused on treating alcoholism. Bill Wilson, the founder of Alcoholics Anonymous, tried LSD and was very impressed with its ability to open up a direct connection to God, self, and the cosmos. Recognizing that such profound spiritual epiphanies could provide a lifeline for others struggling with alcoholism, he enthusiastically endorsed its use. But his organization's leadership, understandably skeptical of substance-based solutions, expressed grave concern, and Wilson gave up his self-experiments.

At the same time, the U. S. government investigated LSD as a potential mind control agent. In 1953, the CIA introduced Project MKUltra, a program that examined the effectiveness of LSD, as well as hypnosis, sensory deprivation, and psychological torture, in brainwashing and incapacitating unsuspecting victims. Over the program's twenty years of operation, the agency illegally dosed hundreds of mental patients, prison inmates, students, and others with LSD, all without their consent or knowledge. Unsurprisingly, adverse reactions were common. One CIA researcher, Frank Olson, suffered a mental breakdown in the days after being unwittingly dosed, and fell—or jumped—out of a hotel window to his death. LSD rarely leads to such dangerous behavior when taken intentionally, but when people are dosed without their knowledge, its effects are much more unpredictable.

TURN ON, TUNE IN, DROP OUT

LSD did not truly come into its own until the 1960s, an era with which it is still indelibly linked. The time was ripe for upheaval, and there was little that LSD didn't touch. Before the decade was through, politics, spirituality, popular music, art, literature, sexuality, and psychiatry would all be upended by the compound's brain-bending effects.

Scientific research continued to flourish, examining the compound's usefulness in treating neurosis, chronic pain, and opioid addiction, as well as anxiety in cancer patients. Realizing that psychedelics could help more than just the sick, scientists also began investigating LSD's ability to foster creativity and problem-solving skills in healthy volunteers.

On the East Coast, Timothy Leary—a professor at Harvard who oversaw the university's psilocybin research program until he was fired in 1963—quickly emerged as the compound's most vocal advocate. He began speaking at counter-cultural events, such as San Francisco's Human Be-In in 1967, where he coined the phrase, "Turn on, tune in, drop out," a mantra encouraging countercultural rebels to detach themselves from the rat race of modern society and get high in the name of spiritual development. His unrestrained—some say reckless—endorsement of LSD would lead President Nixon to brand him, "the most danger-ous man in America," and later led to a cultural backlash against psychedelics.

Meanwhile, on the West Coast, San Francisco was quickly emerging as the psychedelic epicenter of the world. In 1967's Summer of Love, an estimated one hundred thousand hippies from around the country descended on the city's Haight-Ashbury district, spreading a message of peace, love, and anticonsumerism. LSD was available in spades, though the state of California had banned it a year earlier.

LSD was regarded as the wunderkind of psychiatry.

Sixty miles (96.5 km) south of San Francisco in sunny La Honda, Ken Kesey, the author of *One Flew Over the Cuckoo's Nest*, established himself as the ringleader of a ragtag group called the Merry Pranksters. The Pranksters became famous for hosting wild parties featuring outlandish visual displays and endless pitchers of LSD-laced Kool-Aid. Live music came courtesy of Kesey's favorite band, a then-unknown group called the Grateful Dead.

The Merry Pranksters' best-known exploit—immortalized in Tom Wolfe's famous account, *The Electric Kool-Aid Acid Test*—was their 1964 cross-country voyage in an outrageously painted bus named Further. The Pranksters hosted impromptu parties along the way, handing out hits of acid to anyone courageous enough to join the festivities.

In 1965, the Grateful Dead started gaining traction among acid fans and hippies. Before long, an entire subculture of "Deadheads" coalesced around them: For several decades, Grateful Dead shows served as a de facto LSD distribution network. In fact, the group's original audio engineer and financier, Owsley Stanley, was a skilled chemist who produced massive quantities of acid. In two years alone he produced more than five million doses of the stuff, leading *Rolling Stone* magazine to dub him the "king of LSD."

"THE MOST BEAUTIFUL DEATH"
OF ALDOUS HUXLEY

Aldous Huxley, whose writings left a tremendous influence on psychedelic culture, died in 1963. On his deathbed, unable to speak, he scrawled a note asking his wife, Laura, to administer 100 micrograms of LSD by syringe. She obliged, and, a few hours later, with Laura encouraging him, "up and toward the light," he passed away.

Laura Huxley later wrote that it had been, "the most serene, the most beautiful death. Both doctors and nurse said they had never seen a person in similar physical condition going off so completely without pain and without struggle." Aldous Huxley, who had written so convincingly of the value of psychedelics in his books, ended his own story in a state of LSD-infused tranquility—true to his ideals to the very last.

THE END OF AN ERA

LSD's golden age was not to last. As antidrug hysteria mounted and government officials became increasingly alarmed, the tides of public opinion turned firmly against the psychedelic instigator. In 1966, it was banned in California. Federal prohibition followed two years later, and production and distribution went underground.

It was the end of an era, but the beginning of a new one. A number of chemists and distributors took up the charge of getting LSD to the masses. They differed from the stereotypical drug dealer in at least one major way: They believed their product had a positive effect on the world, and that by breaking the law, they could genuinely change humanity for the better. This was the attitude of Nick Sand and Tim Scully, the clandestine chemists responsible for the era's most iconic and well-loved acid "brand," Orange Sunshine.

Though he was LSD's greatest champion, Timothy Leary unwittingly helped hammer the nails in its coffin. Modern researchers point to Leary's irresponsible promotion of drug use as a key reason for the substance's prohibition, effectively shutting down scientific research for decades.

Rampant stories about flashbacks, "acid casualties," and misinformation about its health risks all dented LSD's sterling reputation. The most alarming cases—people throwing themselves off rooftops in an attempt to fly or someone going permanently insane and insisting they were a glass of orange juice—can be chalked up to urban legends and willful deceptions spread by antidrug crusaders. Most health scares, such as the belief that LSD remains in the body for years or caused chromosomal damage and birth defects, were completely unfounded.

Nevertheless, there are real risks to tripping, and some of the "burnout" stories contain a glimmer of truth. Hallucinogen persisting perceptual disorder (HPPD) is now recognized as a very rare condition where the visual effects linger for months or years after the trip ends. LSD and other psychedelics are also believed to exacerbate mental illnesses such as schizophrenia, so today's researchers carefully screen out subjects with a history of such conditions.

Hoping to avoid a repeat of the Leary-era backlash to psychedelics, modern consciousness researchers tread cautiously. Early research produced promising results in a broad range of applications, but was frequently compromised by poor methodology—something contemporary researchers have been eager to amend.

A few scientists brave enough to resurrect this revolutionary chemical have hit upon groundbreaking results. Perhaps one of the greatest findings is the simple fact that, in a controlled and supportive environment, LSD can be safely administered with very few "bad trips" or adverse physical reactions. This helps assuage

INTRODUCING
THE MICRODOSE

Psychedelics are famous for producing intense emotional journeys, but the relatively new phenomenon of "microdosing" turns that on its head. A microdose is one-twentieth to one-tenth of a normal dose of LSD, or another psychedelic, taken once every few days with the aim of improving mood, creativity, and general well-being. The dose is far too small to send one on a trippy voyage, but just enough to bring a certain "lift" to one's daily activities. Showing up to work on acid might sound like a terrible idea, but advocates of microdosing claim it actually improves focus and performance. Supposedly, even Albert Hofmann indulged in the occasional LSD microdose and argued the "subperceptual" dose was an understudied aspect of psychedelics.

The microdosing trend has exploded in popularity in recent years, especially in the psychedelic hotbed of San Francisco. Silicon Valley techies, writers, artists, and thousands of other people around the world have shared anecdotes about the benefits of microdosing in recent years, but science is just catching up. A new study enrolling more than 1,500 respondents found a number of tentative but promising results. Migraine sufferers report their headaches are greatly reduced in intensity and duration. Students report improved grades and better focus, and some women who had experienced painful or emotionally troubling periods report healthy, pain-free cycles. Others indicate improvements in their relationships, a greater sense of openness and gratitude, and reductions in depression. The self-reported benefits have not yet been tested in a strict scientific setting to eliminate placebo effects, but they suggest avenues of future research. And best of all, because doses are so low, adverse effects are practically unheard of.

the lingering drug hysteria from previous decades and opens the door for further therapeutic studies.

Starting in the early 1970s, LSD research stopped cold for more than forty years. In 2014, MAPS (Multidisciplinary Association for Psychedelic Studies) published a study triumphantly breaking the silence. It showed that when combined with talk therapy, LSD reduced anxiety in patients with terminal illnesses. Death-related anxiety is exceptionally difficult to treat. Because its origins are existential rather than chemical, traditional medications offer little solace. LSD-assisted psychotherapy provided relief for the majority of subjects; as patients grappled with their own mortality, they emerged with a new perspective on death, intent on maximizing the value of their remaining days. It was a lasting peace; twelve months later, surviving patients still showed reduced anxiety and improved quality of life.

In 2016, researchers at London's Imperial College produced the first-ever brain scans of people tripping on LSD. The images—analyzing both blood flow and electrical activity in different regions of the brain—showed an expanded state of visualization, even while subjects remained in a dark MRI machine with their eyes closed. According to the study's authors, Dr. David Nutt and Dr. Robin Carhart-Harris, the visual cortex became much more connected to disparate parts of the brain than in sober consciousness.

Another effect, which rose and fell in concert with subjects' reports of "ego dissolution" and feelings of oneness with their environment, was the dampening of what's known as the default mode network (DMN)—a widely distributed group of neurons that fire together while the brain is at rest, not focusing on any particular task. According to Nutt and Carhart-Harris, their results show this network is at least partly responsible for the sense of self we call the "ego." LSD appears to produce its famous boundary-blurring effects by reducing coordination between neurons in the DMN. So LSD's "mind-expanding" effects are due to overall greater "crosstalk" between brain regions that usually remain isolated. By quieting the role of the ego, LSD produces a more connected—albeit more chaotic—brain.

Early research often focused on LSD's potential in treating alcoholism. A 2012 meta-analysis of six of the best studies from that era, consisting of more than five hundred total subjects, found that acid does in fact reduce problematic drinking, at least short term. A single dose significantly reduced alcohol abuse for several months afterward.

Another condition that's notoriously difficult to treat is cluster headaches, which cause excruciating pain. A 2006 study found that, for 80 percent of a small group of people suffering from cluster headaches, LSD eliminated their headaches and extended the period between them. Five years later, a second study showed that 2-Bromo-LSD—a derivative first developed by Albert Hofmann—may be just as effective, without producing any of the psychedelic symptoms of its more famous namesake.

A flurry of other studies have produced interesting results. A 2015 study found no link between mental health problems and the use of LSD and psilocybin in 19,000 randomly selected psychedelic users. Another study in the same year found that people on LSD produced feelings of "happiness, trust, closeness to others, [and] . . . emotional empathy," while impairing the ability to recognize sad and fearful faces. Yet another 2015 study—coauthored by Dr. Carhart-Harris, who produced the first LSD brain scans—demonstrated the compound's ability to increase creative imagination and suggestibility. That won't surprise anyone who's tried acid, but it may prove medically relevant as suggestibility has proved helpful in treating conditions like chronic pain and depression.

Two recent studies demonstrated a heightened emotional response to music. In the first, people's reactions to music featured especially high ratings of "wonder," "transcendence," "power," and "tenderness." In the second study, conducted in Switzerland in 2017, researchers teased apart a fundamental aspect of human consciousness: the attribution of meaning. When sober, people listened to selections of "free jazz" music and found it unengaging. On LSD, they not only found the music pleasant and personally meaningful, but described instances of synesthesia, such as hearing colors and seeing sounds. The substance not only enhances our emotional sensitivity, but allows us to perceive deep personal meaning where none existed before.

Albert Hofmann was heartened by the resurgence of research. Before he died in 2008, at the ripe age of 102, he witnessed the beginning of LSD's rehabilitation in science and public opinion. He had watched his creation, which he dubbed his "problem child," come full circle—from an unexpected but promising birth, through a worrying adolescence of excess and abandon, and finally to the first signs of an adulthood rooted in moderation and rationality.

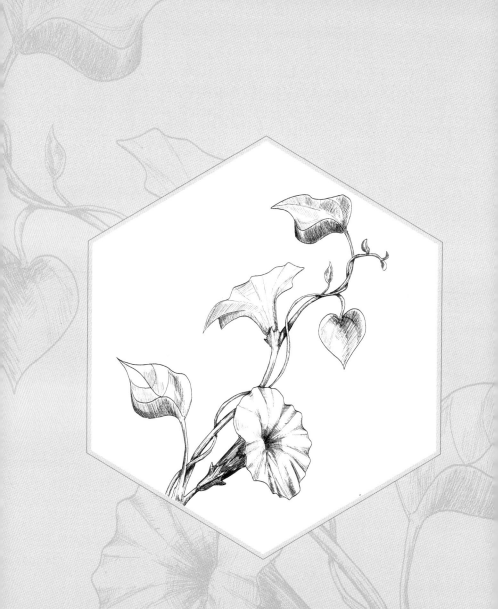

FIG. 1.7

TURBINA CORYMBOSA (SHOWN), *IPOMOEA TRICOLOR, ARGYREIA NERVOSA,*
AND OTHERS

MORNING GLORY

ASSOCIATED WITH *the Aztecs, Maya, and native tribes of Mexico*

KEY COMPOUNDS *ergine (LSA), isoergine, methergine*

ORIGINS AND BACKGROUND

To a gardener, morning glories are a beautiful and sprawling plant, with sprays of brilliant indigo flowers sprouting off vines that wind themselves around anything they touch. But to pre-Columbian civilizations such as the Aztecs, these charming climbers served as a primary visionary plant. Among some indigenous peoples in Mexico, they're still used today for divination and healing.

In the sixteenth century, these visionary substances rubbed the Spanish authorities the wrong way. Unable to honor or integrate the sacramental plants they encountered in the New World, the Spaniards opted to suppress them. Like peyote and psilocybin mushrooms, the secret of *ololiuhqui*—the name of the seeds in Nahuatl, the native tongue of the Aztecs—was nearly lost to time. What the Native Americans saw as a sacrosanct tradition was, to the Spanish invaders, nothing but "satanic hallucinations." By the early twentieth century, there was doubt over whether morning glory seeds were psychoactive at all. (One imagines a simple trial would have put that question to rest.)

But like the vines on which they grew, ololiuhqui proved tenacious, winding furtively through the centuries to find sunlight in the present day. What once was a punishable secret under Spanish rule has now become a common fact: Morning glory seeds offer passage into realms of higher consciousness.

As word got out, the old Aztec sacrament spread far beyond the borders of Mexico. Seen by many as a legal LSD surrogate, the seeds of morning glories—

and of a related species, the Hawaiian Baby Woodrose—have earned a newfound popularity among those looking for psychedelic euphoria without the legal woes.

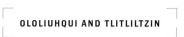

OLOLIUHQUI AND TLITLILTZIN

There are more than one thousand members of Convolvulaceae, the morning glory family, yet only a few are prized for their high concentration of psychoactive components.

Among the Maya and Aztecs, two species reigned supreme. *Ololiuhqui*, which means "round thing," refers to the rounded, brown seeds of *Turbina corymbosa*, whose flowers are white and bell-shaped. *Tlitliltzin*, however, refers to the elongated black seeds of *Ipomea tricolor*, whose flowers sport a pinwheel of blue petals around a white and gold center. The Zapotec, Mazatec, and Mixtec tribes still use these seeds today in divination and healing ceremonies. Like their ancestors, modern shamans prepare the seeds by grinding them to a fine powder and preparing a cold tea.

The Aztecs had a more unusual use for the seeds. Aztec boys would collect venomous creatures, including spiders, scorpions, and snakes, burn them to ashes, and mix the powder with ground tobacco and ololiuhqui. The resulting dark paste was "placed in vessels and cups before their god like divine food." Aztec priests even smeared the ooze upon their bodies to commune with their gods.

Among the native peoples of Oaxaca, the use of morning glory seeds presents a stark contrast to other New World entheogens, such as peyote and psilocybin mushrooms. Unlike these better-known visionary substances, ololiuhqui is usually taken in solitary settings, in a quiet location with only the shaman and—when healing is sought—the afflicted individual.

SPAIN AND THE SNAKE PLANT

Europe first encountered psychedelic morning glory seeds in the sixteenth century, when Spain conquered the Aztecs. Dr. Francisco Hernández, court physician of the king of Spain, reported on the appearance and medicinal qualities of the plant, describing it as a "twining herb" with "long white flowers." The natives, he said, called the vine *coaxihuitl*, meaning "snake plant."

Hernández sang its praises as a cure-all. He recommended it as a remedy for syphilis, pain, and even excessive "flatulency." Prepared as a poultice, it was said to be good for chills, dislocations, fractures, eye diseases, and "pelvic troubles for women." As a drink, it was a potent aphrodisiac.

About those "pelvic troubles," Hernández was surprisingly correct. Ergometrine and methylergometrine, two compounds found in morning glory seeds, have become mainstays of modern obstetrics. They cause contractions of the uterus and are widely used to treat excessive bleeding in postpartum women. For the same reason, pregnant women should never take morning glory seeds in a nonmedical context. More recently, methylergometrine has also shown considerable promise in treating migraine headaches.

About its psychological effects, Hernández was less glowing. He wrote, "When the priests wanted to commune with their gods and to receive a message from them, they ate this plant to induce a delirium. A thousand visions and satanic hallucinations appeared to them." Writing in 1591, Juan de Cárdenas captured the general Spanish attitude toward the hallucinogen. Morning glory seeds, he wrote, "will cause the wretch who takes them to lose his wits so severely that he sees the devil among other terrible and fearsome apparitions."

In retrospect, it appears that the Spaniards, not the natives, were afflicted with demonic hallucinations; where the conquered tribesmen found serenity and understanding, the Spainiards saw devils.

Consuming the seeds is a serious matter. The natives enter into the ololiuhqui trance in the manner of pilgrims approaching a sacred temple—quiet, deferential, and seeking answers to pressing questions, such as the nature of an illness or the will of the ancestors.

A BOTANICAL DISPUTE

Though scholars had identified ololiuhqui as a morning glory species as early as 1854, the hallucinogen's true identity was disputed for many years. It was

Morning glories have earned a newfound popularity among those looking for psychedelic euphoria without the legal woes.

Richard Evans Schultes who finally settled the matter. Having observed its use by Zapotec medicine men, Schultes collected samples of *Turbina corymbosa* and sent them to Albert Hofmann, the chemist who had discovered LSD.

Hofmann's analysis revealed that the plant contained ergot alkaloids—substances closely related to LSD. This was an unexpected—and heavily scrutinized— revelation, as these chemicals had previously been discovered only in ergot, a fungus totally unrelated to the morning glory family. Some remained skeptical, but later analyses bore out his findings. Hofmann proved that morning glories were the first—and so far only—plant family to contain lysergic acid compounds.

No one knows exactly which compounds are responsible for the seeds' remarkable effects. Psychoactive effects may result from the intermingling of several alkaloids. It is commonly assumed that ergine, also known as LSA, or lysergic acid amide, is the most important compound, but its exact role remains uncertain.

THE EXPERIENCE

The high from morning glory seeds has been compared to LSD, but is often regarded as more placid. The cocktail of lysergic chemicals in the seeds is less stimulating than their more famous cousin and has even been called sedating. Nausea is extremely common, but often passes after vomiting.

Dr. Humphry Osmond, a British-born psychiatrist who introduced Aldous Huxley to mescaline, became curious about these hotly debated seeds. In 1955, he engaged in a series of self-experiments. On the first few occasion, the seeds had little effect. But his later experiences—with sixty and then one hundred seeds, pulverized with a mortar and pestle—were more powerful.

Osmond's terse notes provide a window into the first recorded encounter of a Westerner with the famed Mexican sacrament.

People irritate; things fascinate; the texture of wood; the almost metallic gold center of an African violet. Mildly nauseated. The little warm dog on my lap the only contact.

Overall, he remarked, "irritable apathy" was the hallmark of the experience. He also described a surreal sense of depersonalization and "complete detachment," more typical of dissociatives such as ketamine and PCP.

But it was not altogether unpleasant. A full 11 hours after dosing, Osmond noted there was

> . . . still a depth and brightness in things such as they have on a May morning when you are twenty-one. A newness, freshness as if everything had had a shower.

Osmond's experience may not be typical. Many takers of morning glory and Hawaiian Baby Woodrose seeds have reported all the usual hallmarks of psychedelic experiences: swirling, kaleidoscopic imagery, bizarre physical sensations, emotional sensitivity, and even the breakdown of time and space. Osmond may be the first non-Native American to consume the seeds and report the results, but his experience of "irritable apathy" was hardly definitive.

THE HAWAIIAN BABY WOODROSE

Though the Hawaiian Baby Woodrose is more potent than all other morning glory species, it has never been used as an entheogen by any historical cultures. Its unusually high potency came to light in the latter half of the twentieth century. Though concentrations vary, five seeds of Hawaiian Baby Woodrose are roughly the equivalent of one hundred to one hundred fifty seeds of other species.

Like most of its cousins, *Argyreia nervosa* boasts broad, heart-shaped leaves and bell-like flowers. Unlike typical ornamental varieties, however, the lavender flowers of Hawaiian Baby Woodrose have dark, almost black, centers looking more like watchful pupils than bursts of light.

In spite of its name, the plant is neither Hawaiian nor a rose. In fact, it is native to India, the home of the mysterious *soma* visionary ritual and the birthplace of the cannabis beverage called *bhang*. In a place where even the gods consume cannabis, it's a wonder the psychedelic qualities of such a fetching flowering vine escaped notice for so many centuries. But now that the cat's out of the bag, Hawaiian Baby Woodrose seeds are in high demand among botanically minded trippers. It now grows throughout the tropical regions of the world, including parts of Africa, islands in the Caribbean, and, of course, Hawaii.

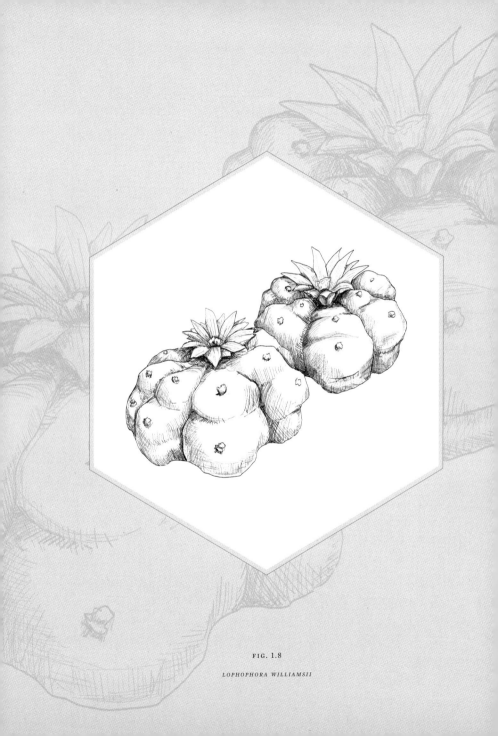

FIG. 1.8

LOPHOPHORA WILLIAMSII

DISCOVERED

Used by indigenous
peoples for more than
six thousand years

PEYOTE

ASSOCIATED WITH *indigenous peoples of Mexico, Aldous Huxley, and the Native American Church*

KEY COMPOUND *mescaline*

ORIGINS AND BACKGROUND

O NE OF HUMANITY'S OLDEST PSYCHEDELIC TRADITIONS, the peyote ritual was already several thousand years old when the Spaniards encountered it in the sixteenth century. The cactus, long revered by natives as a sacred visionary medicine and a central pillar of their way of life—even recognized by some tribes as a deity itself—was viciously suppressed by the invading Spanish forces who had very different views on God and holiness. What the natives saw as the gateway to spirituality, the Conquistadors condemned as a satanic drug scourge.

Since then, peyote has remained a point of tension between native and European peoples in the Americas. Today, despite its prohibited status in the United States, peyote use is permitted for members of the Native American Church. It is one of only two religious sacraments exempt from federal drug laws; the other is ayahuasca (see page 40).

Peyote is native to the deserts of Mexico and southern Texas, where it grows extremely slowly: It can take more than ten years for a plant to reach maturity. Unable to regrow fast enough to keep up with demand, peyote has been overharvested. Luckily, it grows well in greenhouse conditions.

The plant looks innocuous enough—a small, fuzzy green cactus without any spines. The majority of the plant extends underground like a carrot. What remain aboveground are the crowns, which can be cut and cured into "buttons" or mescals for ritual consumption, leaving the plant intact to grow new crowns. Upon each crown, wavy furrows extend outward from the center like twisted spokes, lending a geometric, almost symbolic, look to the humble green bulb. At the center grows a single flower with brilliant pink petals.

Peyote's quaint appearance belies its profound effects on the human mind, which have been utilized for healing and journeying by native peoples for countless generations. It can be consumed raw, dried, or as a bitter tea. The name derives from the Nahuatl *peyotl*, meaning "divine messenger."

Nausea and vomiting are very common in the early stages, and some say peyote gives you the hangover before the experience. This quickly gives way to full-fledged psychedelia, including vivid kaleidoscopic imagery, enhanced empathy, and often-profound spiritual experiences. The effects are reminiscent of psilocybin mushrooms or LSD, but many find peyote milder and less disorienting, perhaps due to the difficulty of choking down more than a handful

THE DISCOVERY OF MESCALINE

Named after the Mescalero, an Apache tribe located in New Mexico, mescaline was the first natural psychedelic compound to be extracted, isolated, and synthesized. Its discovery by German chemist Arthur Heffter in 1897 predated the synthesis of DMT and LSD and the isolation of psilocybin from mushrooms by several decades.

Heffter's discovery was a historic event, representing the first collision of indigenous religious practice—ancient, emotional, and subjective—with modern pharmacology—young, detached, and objective. The intermingling of the religious experience and pharmacology, two seemingly opposite approaches to sacred psychoactive plants, would prove increasingly fruitful over the course of the twentieth century. This line of research would culminate in the finding, first observed at Harvard in 1962, that psychedelics could reliably produce profound mystical states indistinguishable from spontaneous religious experiences.

of the extremely bitter buttons. Overall, a peyote trip takes between 8 and 12 hours. The cactus contains hundreds of alkaloids, but its primary psychedelic constituent is mescaline.

CACTUS CONTRABAND AND RELIGIOUS PERSECUTION IN NEW SPAIN

Peyote has been a friend of humanity's for at least six millennia. In the 1930s, researchers discovered peyote specimens at Shumla Caves, an archaeological site located in southwestern Texas along the Rio Grande River. They confirmed the presence of mescaline and dated the material to around 4000 BCE.

Bernardino de Sahagún, a sixteenth-century missionary priest and dedicated ethnographer, became the first to write of the native peyote customs:

> *It is called Peiotl. It is white. . . . Those who eat or drink it see visions either*
> *frightful or laughable. This intoxication lasts two or three days and then ceases.*
> *It is a common food of the Chichimeca, for it sustains them and gives them courage*
> *to fight and not feel fear nor hunger nor thirst. And they say that*
> *it protects them from all danger.*

The natives used peyote for a variety of purposes, such as finding lost or stolen items, foretelling the future, and healing almost any malady—from fever and sunstroke to headaches and arthritis. Some tribes used it as a salve for burns and wounds and even to improve endurance in footraces and long hunts.

In 1690, Padre José de Ortega gave the first known description of the peyote ritual itself, which to this day involves hours of dancing, singing, and crying as the cactus's ecstatic trance takes hold:

Peyote's quaint appearance belies its profound effects on the human mind.

*Close to the musician was seated the leader of the singing, whose business it was
to mark time. . . . Nearby was placed a tray filled with Peyote, which is a diabolical
root that is ground up and drunk by them so that they may not become weakened
by the exhausting effects of so long a function . . . One after the other, they went
dancing in a ring or marking time with their feet, keeping in the middle the
musician . . . They would dance all night, from five o'clock in the evening to seven
o'clock in the morning, without stopping nor leaving the circle.*

The Spaniards' rigid Catholicism left no room for such "heathen rituals and superstitions" and consuming peyote was declared an egregious sin. To the natives, who had honored peyote as a sacred plant and portal to the divine, it was as though the white invaders had outlawed God Himself.

A tradition of such power and longevity would not die easily and peyote rituals continued in secret. Even as it shrank from public life, peyote continued to expand northward to new territories, winning over indigenous peoples who lived beyond the cactus's natural habitat and had to acquire the contraband by commerce.

Today, the peyote cult extends far beyond the Chihuahuan Desert and is used ceremonially by Apache, Comanche, Navajo, and other tribes stretching across the Great Plains as far north as Canada. Customs vary, but a few factors are common: Gatherings are usually held at night around a blazing bonfire, with much singing and dancing. At the center of the ceremony, of course, is peyote— and the gods and ancestors to whom it offers a direct and powerful communion.

THE HUICHOL

Anthropologists believe the traditions of today's Huichol people bear the closest resemblance to the peyote rites of centuries past. Every year, the Huichol *mara'akame*, or shaman, leads a pilgrimage to the holy land of Wirikuta, three hundred miles (483 km) from their home. He is joined by a group of pilgrims that includes men, women, and children.

Today, any member of the Church may partake in its peyote ceremonies, regardless of ethnicity.

At the sacred grounds, the pilgrims perform a ritualized ceremony and gather peyote to bring back to their people—enough to use for an entire year and to trade to nearby tribes who have no such harvest.

The Huichol are also famous for their vision inspired art, which bursts with spectacular colors and geometric designs. The yarn paintings and beaded objects are now popular as tourist items but are still rooted in the tribe's longstanding aesthetic language. Motifs such as deer, corn, and peyote are rendered in stunning color, interwoven with hypnotic patterns representing the visions induced by the cactus. These psychedelic artworks are also created as offerings and left at mountain shrines and other holy locations to express gratitude to the gods.

NATIVE AMERICAN CHURCH AND THE REVIVAL OF PEYOTE

Persecuted for centuries for practicing their ancestors' way of life on their own land, native peoples banded together in the early twentieth century to spread and protect their peyote practice under the banner of a new institution: the Native American Church. In the latter decades of the 1800s, peyote had already spilled beyond Mexico's borders and gained popularity among tribes that had no historical connection to the cactus.

The Church was incorporated in 1918, combining traditional native spiritual tradition with aspects of Protestant Christianity. Although the Church's membership quickly reached the tens of thousands, all was not well—more than a dozen states outlawed possession of peyote by 1930. A federal ban came in 1970. But the story of peyote is one of persistence, and members of the Native American Church soldiered on just as their predecessors had done under the rule of the Spaniards. In 1994, Congress finally passed a law guaranteeing Native Americans the right to their time-honored sacrament. Today, any member of the Church may partake in its peyote ceremonies, regardless of ethnicity. Science has also helped exonerate the "devil's root." A 2005 study showed that regular peyote use among Navajo members was not linked to any psychological or cognitive deficits.

With more than a quarter million members, the Native American Church is the largest indigenous religion in all of North America. Its loose association of diverse peoples shares a common sacrament in a variety of peyote ceremonies that may commemorate birthdays, Easter, Christmas, and births and deaths. These events are usually held in a teepee or roundhouse with singing and drumming. The peyote is placed on a clay altar, and a bag of dried buttons is passed around to each attendee. And although the Church has many Christian leanings, its members have no need of priests: The peyote itself connects humankind directly to the Great Spirit.

MESCALINE AND WESTERN CULTURE

Peyote and mescaline have spread beyond the confines of Native American communities and have crossed paths with more than a few gringos over the years.

Perhaps the chief mescaline proponent of the twentieth century was Aldous Huxley, whose pioneering 1954 book, *The Doors of Perception*, vividly described his experience with the compound. It quickly became a touchstone in the nascent field of psychedelic literature. By introducing curious Westerners to mescaline, and, more broadly, to the psychedelic experience, Huxley opened the doors of perception for generations of explorers.

Huxley waxed poetic about his first experience with the compound, viewing with fresh eyes, "the miracle, moment by moment, of naked existence." Looking at a bouquet of flowers, he had a realization about what he called "Is-ness" or "Suchness"—the inherent quality of existence that lends all things meaning. "This is how one ought to see, how things really are," he intoned.

A number of musicians have experimented with mescaline, such as members of the Eagles, one of the preeminent bands of the 1970s. Describing a peyote-infused photo shoot of the band in the Mojave Desert, drummer and co-lead singer Don Henley said:

There was a pervasive feeling that we were embarking on a momentous journey; there was an air of portent in the positive sense. It was simultaneously a sensory and a spiritual experience. . . . Under the effects of peyote, in the glowing dusk, we saw the Joshua trees as sentient beings.

Jim Morrison was so enamored of Huxley's *The Doors of Perception* that he borrowed its title for his band, The Doors. Huxley's title was in turn borrowed from a memorable line by the English poet and painter, William Blake:

If the doors of perception were cleansed, everything would appear to man as it is, infinite. For man has closed himself up, till he sees all things thro' narrow chinks of his cavern.

Blake wasn't talking about mescaline, but he may as well have been. The same sentiments have been echoed by the Huichol and other indigenous tribes, who believe this world is illusory. To them, true reality is revealed in the visions granted by the sacred peyote, the great cleanser of the doors of perception.

THE BIRTH OF A WORD

Psychiatrist Humphry Osmond also coined the term *psychedelic* in correspondence with his friend Aldous Huxley. When Osmond asked for a new word to encapsulate visionary substances like psilocybin, LSD, and mescaline, Huxley suggested *phanerothyme*, from the Greek roots for "show" and "spirit":

To make this trivial world sublime, take half a gram of phanerothyme.

Osmond replied with his own proposal, formed from the Greek roots *psyche* (mind) and *deloun* (show or manifest):

To fathom Hell or soar angelic just take a pinch of psychedelic.

The name stuck. Sorry, Aldous, but it's for the best—the "Phanerothymic Sixties" just doesn't have the same ring to it.

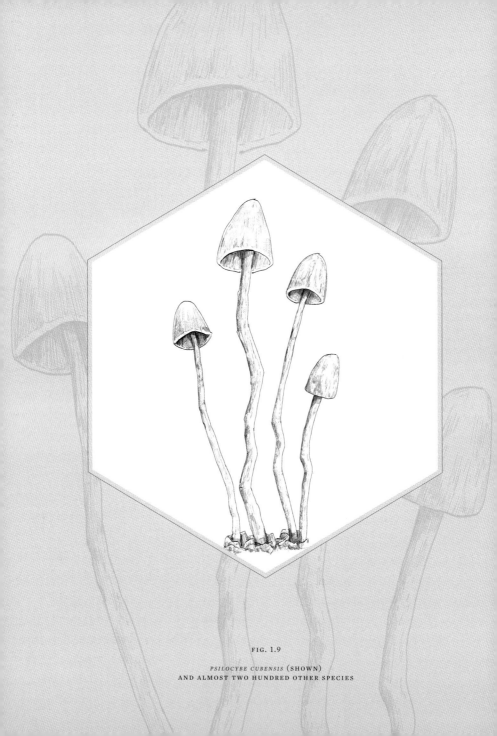

FIG. 1.9

PSILOCYBE CUBENSIS (SHOWN)
AND ALMOST TWO HUNDRED OTHER SPECIES

DISCOVERED

Used by natives in the
Americas for at least
five centuries

PSILOCYBIN MUSHROOMS

ASSOCIATED WITH *Terence McKenna, Timothy Leary*

KEY COMPOUNDS *psilocybin and psilocin*

ORIGINS AND BACKGROUND

KNOWN AS *TEONANÁCATL* TO THE AZTECS, *'nti-si-tho* to the Mazatec, magic mushrooms to the hippies, and simply "shrooms" to the modern enthusiast, psilocybin-containing fungi have many names—and many fans. Today, the humble mushroom is one of the best-known members of the psychedelic family, represented by hundreds of species growing all across the world. So it's hard to believe they were once a well-guarded secret known only to a handful of native peoples in Central America. Their very existence was doubted by top anthropologists and biologists until recently, thanks to a centuries-long campaign by Spanish invaders to stamp out the "demonic" mushrooms.

The Catholic authorities were ultimately unsuccessful. Today, no one doubts the existence of these little toadstools, nor their incredible power. The mushrooms have returned in full force, and their active components, psilocybin and psilocin, are shaking up the worlds of neuroscience and medicine.

The quaint mushrooms and the mystical realms they unlock have a universal and timeless appeal. From the mountains of Mexico to the halls of Harvard, from the centuries before Christ to the age of the Internet, for shamans and healers, professors, reverends and inmates, psilocybin has shifted perspectives and granted vistas of vast new worlds within.

The effects of psilocybin mushrooms last between 3 and 6 hours and produce a wide range of sensory and emotional distortions ranging from animated visual patterns to deep personal insights. For many, mushrooms represent the definitive psychedelic experience.

Changes to the senses become apparent within 30 minutes of ingestion. Textures and patterns drift through the air, melting into arabesques and undulating geometries. Colors become impossibly rich, memories come alive with the vitality of the present moment, words and faces are imbued with an unfathomable poignancy, and the ears open up as if for the first time, revealing previously ignored details in the sonic landscape.

Often, traumas and insecurities bubble to the surface of one's consciousness. If the user is prepared to confront and sit with them, profound healing is possible; if not, the trip may take a dark and unpleasant turn. A handbook used in psychedelic therapy sessions encourages subjects to embrace difficult feelings, even if the first instinct is to recoil: "Look for the darkest corner in the basement, and shine your light there."

With the right dosage and setting, psilocybin is well known for providing mystical experiences characterized by the dissolution of one's sense of self, leaving only a boundless impression of cosmic unity and bliss. Reports of encounters with God, spirits, or benevolent forces are common. Those lucky enough to experience such a state often rank it as one of the most meaningful moments of their lives.

MUSHROOMS IN ANCIENT HISTORY

Varieties of psilocybin mushrooms grow all over the world, but today their traditional use is limited to just a few neighboring tribes in southern Mexico. Evidence on prehistoric use is scant, but it appears religious mushroom consumption was once more widespread—and has been occurring for thousands of years. In Guatemala, hundreds of carved mushroom stones dot the countryside, dating back to the Maya civilization three thousand years ago. Each stone features a stylized figure, such as a human, bird, or toad, capped by a rounded dome resembling a cartoonish mushroom. The function of these mushroom stones remains a mystery, but some anthropologists are convinced that the Maya, like the Aztecs two millennia later, used psilocybin mushrooms in religious settings and held them in very high esteem.

Cave paintings at Tassili n'Ajjer in northwestern Algeria, dating from 5000 to 7000 BCE, depict psychedelic mushroom consumption. In one, a group of human figures with mushroomlike caps appears to race down a hill, mushrooms in hand. Dotted lines connect each mushroom to its holder's head, as if to indicate a connection between the fungus and the runner's mind. In another, a shaman wearing a beelike mask is portrayed with mushrooms sprouting from every surface of his body and bursting forth from between his fingers. *Psilocybe mairei* grows in Algeria and may have been available to the muralists. The question remains whether the artists worked with fungal inspiration.

THE CONQUISTADORS VERSUS THE MUSHROOM

When the Spaniards conquered the Aztec empire in the beginning of the sixteenth century, they learned of three psychedelic species held in high esteem by the natives: the peyote cactus, morning glory seeds, and hallucinogenic mushrooms. The Aztecs prized the latter in particular, calling them *teonanácatl* or "divine mushrooms." Where the Aztecs saw God, however, the Spaniards perceived only the nefarious work of the devil.

"When they are eaten or drunk," wrote one missionary, "they intoxicate, depriving those who partake of them of their senses and making them believe a thousand absurdities."

King Phillip II's personal doctor, Francisco Hernández, reported that one type of mushroom causes mainly "unconditional laughter." Others "bring before the eyes all kinds of visions, such as wars and the likeness of demons." The natives' nightlong mushroom ceremonies, he said, were both "terrifying and awesome."

Where the Aztecs saw God, the Spaniards perceived only the nefarious work of the devil.

A Franciscan friar described how the indigenous peoples hallucinated "a thousand visions, especially snakes. They went raving mad, and they ran about the streets wildly."

Devils and demons, snakes and beasts, scenes of violence and depravity—the Spaniards projected all manner of dark and menacing visions upon the mysterious mushrooms. Throughout time, man has sought to banish whatever frightens or perplexes him, and the Catholic authorities carried out their duty with great relish. The way of the mushroom did not die, but it went deep underground.

For four centuries, the mushrooms remained little more than a legend. The native peoples' religious, medicinal, and celebratory mushroom traditions all but evaporated from the historical record. But indigenous peoples must have continued to practice the way of their ancestors in secret, passing the knowledge from one generation to the next. How else to explain the unlikely reappearance of the mushrooms, nearly half a millennium later, among indigenous people in the Mexican state of Oaxaca?

THE WEST DISCOVERS MUSHROOMS—AGAIN

"Magic" mushrooms remained unknown to Europeans throughout most of modern history, only breaking into popular consciousness in the twentieth century. In 1938, Richard Evans Schultes, the great Harvard scholar and explorer of the Amazon, and Dr. Blas Pablo Reko, an Austrian botanist, visited the Mazatec tribe in northeastern Oaxaca, where the natives showed them something few white men had ever seen—the sacred mushrooms. Samples were identified as various species of the genus *Psilocybe*. Still, very little was known about the mushrooms and their ceremonial use until an unlikely champion emerged.

In 1955, banker and amateur mycologist R. Gordon Wasson traveled to Mexico with a friend, where they became "the first white men in recorded history to eat the divine mushrooms." In a feature article published two years later in *Life* magazine, Wasson wrote about his personal experience eating the mushrooms and their ceremonial use by the Mazatec people as an agent of healing and prophesying. A *Life* editor coined the term "magic mushrooms."

The essay exposed the American public to a natural, nontoxic, and easily grown psychedelic that had long been overlooked. Wasson's testimony also showed that such compounds had a long history of spiritual and therapeutic use and were not just for reckless hedonists. As the starry-eyed hippies of the '60s had no other guidance for taking mushrooms, this ceremonial context set a valuable precedent.

Today, everyone knows about "magic mushrooms," and you can order a grow kit to your door in a matter of minutes. But back in 1957, most of the world knew nothing about these furtive fungi. Wasson's adventures brought him to the doorstep of a state of consciousness never before explored by Westerners.

MARÍA SABINA'S
"LITTLE CHILDREN"

R. Gordon Wasson's story in *Life* profoundly influenced the psychedelic movement of the 1960s and led many people to visit María Sabina, the Mazatec healer who had shared the secret of the mushroom with him. After reading the article, Timothy Leary traveled to Mexico and had his own mushroom experience, which ignited his journey as psychedelic researcher and countercultural icon. If it weren't for Wasson's expedition, "shrooms" may have remained an obscure mystery, and Timothy Leary may never have become a household name.

In the next decade, thousands of other spiritual tourists, including Bob Dylan, John Lennon, and Mick Jagger, all descended upon Sabina's village in the hopes of tasting the divine mushroom. Even the chemist Albert Hofmann visited, offering the healer a bottle of pure psilocybin pills. María Sabina sampled them and agreed the experience was much the same as that afforded by her "little children." It wasn't all good news for the traditional Mazatec community, however—the village became thronged with gringos, and María Sabina eventually came to regret serving the mushrooms to foreigners.

PSILOCYBIN RESEARCH

Psilocybin research trailed far behind that of LSD in the 1950s and '60s, but it did garner its share of groundbreaking studies. After the mushrooms' prohibition in 1970, research halted for decades, but psilocybin is now emerging as the cornerstone of contemporary psychedelic research. Today, it's being examined for its role in treating anxiety and alcoholism, helping people quit smoking, and other uses.

One of the first tasks was to isolate the active components that made the mushrooms "magic." Samples were sent to Albert Hofmann, the Swiss chemist who had discovered LSD in 1943. Hofmann identified two serotonin-like compounds responsible for the mushrooms' remarkable mental effects and named them after the genus *Psilocybe*: psilocybin and psilocin.

THE HARVARD PSILOCYBIN PROJECT

In the summer of 1960, Timothy Leary, a promising new lecturer in Harvard's psychology department, had his first taste of psilocybin mushrooms. He found himself, "swept over the edge of a sensory Niagara into a maelstrom of transcendental visions and hallucinations," and later described the event as, "without question the deepest religious experience of [his] life."

When he returned to the university that fall, Leary was a changed man. With the help of his colleague Richard Alpert, another rising star of the Harvard faculty, Leary proposed an innovative research program to investigate psilocybin with human subjects. Thus was born the Harvard Psilocybin Project.

The program would end abruptly three years later, with both Leary and Alpert dismissed amid concerns about the safety, propriety, and legitimacy of the research. But during its short tenure, the Harvard Psilocybin Project enrolled hundreds of curious graduate students, faculty, and even prison inmates in some of the most influential—if deeply flawed—psychedelic studies of the twentieth century.

CONCORD PRISON EXPERIMENT

After his own mushroom experience, Timothy Leary had no doubt about psilocybin's ability to transform people's lives for the better. What better population for testing his theory than hardened criminals? Leary arranged to administer psilocybin to thirty-two inmates of Concord Prison, a maximum-security facility outside Boston, to see if the experience would reduce recidivism and induce positive changes in the inmates' attitudes.

Ever the iconoclast, Leary also insisted the research staff take psilocybin *with* the inmates, to eliminate the power dichotomy of researcher/subject and authority/inmate, instead placing everyone on equal footing as human beings. And that's exactly what they did: In group sessions held in the gray confines of the prison's infirmary, armed with only a record player, tape recorder, and pure psilocybin pills, Leary and his colleagues got trippy with convicted criminals in the name of science.

Leary was thrilled about the results. He claimed he'd cut recidivism by half— a truly monumental feat—but a long-term follow-up study conducted by Rick Doblin identified numerous flaws of the original study, casting serious doubt on its supposed success. Leary had used data misleadingly to paint a rosy picture of psilocybin's effects. In fact, the experimental subjects demonstrated an average rate of recidivism.

Nevertheless, the Concord Prison Experiment remains an indelible part of the story of psychedelics.

GOOD FRIDAY EXPERIMENT

The other historic study from Leary's time at Harvard is known as the Good Friday Experiment. Led by psychiatrist and minister Walter Pahnke, the study examined whether psilocybin could produce "mystical" or religious experiences. Psychedelic researcher Roland Griffiths would later describe the mystical state of consciousness as, "a profound sense of the interconnectedness of all things packaged in a benevolent framework of a sense of sacredness, deep reverence, openhearted love, and a noetic quality of truth."

On Good Friday 1962, Pahnke gathered twenty volunteers from a local seminary school and led them to a sanctuary in the basement of a chapel. The day's service was piped into the room so the students could follow along. Half the theology students received psilocybin; the other half received a placebo with no psychoactive effects.

Within a few minutes, the "active" subjects sprawled out in the pews and on the floor, crying out about the glory of God, while the "placebo" subjects thumbed their Bibles and looked on with raised eyebrows.

Nevertheless, the results were astounding. Almost all the students who had received psilocybin had profound religious experiences, characterized by a sense of unity, transcendence of time and space, and a powerful impression of sacredness. For many, it was a life-changing day, forever altering their understanding of God and spirituality.

In a follow-up study conducted twenty-five years later, all interviewees in the active dose group indicated the experience had affected their lives in significant

SET AND SETTING

The nature of a psychedelic trip depends on what Timothy Leary described as the user's "set and setting." "Set" refers to mind-set, including attitudes, expectations for the trip, and general sense of well-being. Tripping while depressed, anxious, or sleep deprived is a recipe for a difficult journey.

"Setting" refers to one's environment—both the physical surroundings and the emotional tenor of the other people in the room. Journeying with others requires a firm foundation of trust. The psychic risks depend very much on the user's preparedness, a fact confirmed in scientific research by the remarkably few "freak-out" incidents when psychedelics are taken with clear intentions in the company of a trusted therapist.

The idea wasn't totally original, of course. Indigenous peoples have recognized the importance of intention and ritual in the context of psychedelics for many centuries. Leary's accomplishment was in bringing that wisdom to the culture of modern psychology. Instead of the austere hospitals and laboratories used by earlier researchers, Leary opted for comfortable, homey environments—a method echoed in psychedelic research today.

and positive ways. One participant, a future reverend, summarized the experiment succinctly. "We took such an infinitesimal amount of psilocybin, and yet it connected me to infinity."

MODERN RESEARCH

For many years, psychedelic research evaporated entirely. In 2006, a study led by Roland Griffiths at Johns Hopkins University began to reverse that trend. Dr. Griffiths chose to revisit the same question that had motivated the Good Friday Experiment many years earlier: Can psilocybin produce religious experiences? Griffiths found that not only did psilocybin induce "mystical-type" experiences but such experiences carried profound meaning that continued far beyond the original study's duration. More than a year later, subjects ranked their experience on psilocybin as one of the most "personally meaningful and spiritually significant" events of their lives. In another study conducted by Griffiths in 2011, volunteers reported a range of beneficial effects after psilocybin sessions, including lasting improvements to their attitude, mood, and behavior.

Another study found that psilocybin-induced mystical experiences resulted in long-term changes to one of the fundamental aspects of personality, "openness." When this basic personality trait—encompassing one's curiosity, preference for variety, tendency to fantasy, aesthetic sensitivity, and attentiveness to internal feelings—was measured, subjects scored higher for more than a year after a psilocybin-induced mystical experience. This marked the first time in the history of psychology that a single event had caused lasting changes in one of the foundational domains of human personality.

For neuroscientists, psilocybin has proved to be a useful tool that not only produces novel effects but helps shed light on how our brains normally function. In a study led by Robin Carhart-Harris at London's Imperial College, brain scans taken during a psilocybin experience revealed patterns of activity that resembled the dreaming mind. The results demonstrated for the first time the physical underpinnings of the surreal and often dreamlike fantasias revealed by psilocybin.

It has long been assumed that "mind-expanding" substances act by increasing brain activity. But in a groundbreaking 2012 study, brain scans of volunteers tripping on psilocybin revealed the exact opposite. In fact, the compound *reduced* activity in several of the brain's key connective hubs.

This led to greater communication between normally unrelated regions of the brain. These changes were closely associated with the subjective experience of "ego dissolution," where one's sense of self melts into a boundless oceanic state. Psilocybin appears to produce at least some of its effects by inhibiting the parts of the brain responsible for maintaining the ego, unlocking what Dr. Carhart-Harris calls, "a state of unconstrained cognition."

A MEDICINE FOR THE DYING

In addition to its evolving role in spirituality and neuroscience, psilocybin has shown promise as a medicine for a surprising variety of illnesses.

In a 2011 pilot study of people with advanced-stage cancer, lead researcher Dr. Charles Grob turned his attention to one of humankind's most profound and persistent challenges: despair in the face of death. After a single session of psilocybin where they were encouraged to focus on their inward experience, the cancer patients experienced relief from their crippling anxiety. Two 2016 studies confirmed the results, showing that psilocybin reduced both anxiety and depression in cancer patients, with subjects reporting reduced feelings of hopelessness, higher quality of life, and "improved spiritual well-being." In all three studies, the benefits persisted for more than six months.

Because it is rooted in our fear of death itself, the psychological stress associated with terminal diseases is notoriously difficult to treat. Far from an escapist drug, psilocybin appears to help people come to terms with death, helping them reframe their attitudes in a profound way. Any medicine that relieves the suffering of the dying ought to be pursued with great interest.

Psilocybin may even have a preventive effect on suicide. In an analysis of more than two hundred thousand responses to the National Survey on Drug

Use and Health, Peter Hendricks found that people who had used psychedelics were significantly less likely to experience recent psychological distress, suicide attempts, or suicidal thinking. No other class of drugs was associated with improvements in mental health. A causal link has not been established—psychedelic use may be correlated with good mental health without causing it directly—but, hopefully, further research will untangle the results.

DEPRESSION, DEPENDENCE, AND MORE

One unexpected application for psilocybin is in treating stubborn cases of obsessive-compulsive disorder, or OCD. A small 2006 study showed that a single dose of psilocybin could reduce treatment-resistant OCD symptoms for more than 24 hours. Even very low doses caused impressive reductions in obsessive thinking. A small but promising study led by Robin Carhart-Harris showed significant improvements for twelve volunteers with treatment-resistant depression. One week after their session, two-thirds of the participants showed complete remission; at three months, nearly half remained depression free.

Depression is a widespread, complex, and often crippling condition that can be very difficult to treat. Typical treatment approaches combine talk therapy with medications such as Prozac or Zoloft, which must be taken daily and often cause unpleasant side effects, such as emotional blunting. In this small preliminary study, people who had not found relief from any traditional treatments showed substantial and sustained effects after just two doses of psilocybin.

A 2017 study led by the same scientists confirmed these effects while offering new clues to the mechanism behind them. The researchers administered two doses of psilocybin one week apart to nineteen individuals with treatment-resistant depression, taking a baseline brain scan before the first dose and another on the day after the final dose. The majority of subjects experienced rapid improvements in their depression, and several spoke of feeling "reset," as if their brain had been rebooted—results that correlated with what the researchers observed in the brain scans.

When the subjects were presented with images of happy and fearful faces on the day after their final experience, they showed an increased response in the amygdala, a brain region known to process fear and stress. This reaction closely correlated with mood improvements one week later. It appears that psilocybin elicits its antidepressant effects by fostering a powerful emotional reconnection—in stark contrast to traditional antidepressants, which dull the response of the amygdala and often have a blunting effect on emotions.

The results remain to be confirmed by larger, more rigorous studies. But if this mushroom ingredient can cure the most stubborn cases of depression in a matter of weeks, replacing a whole medicine cabinet of "maintenance drugs" with one or two peak experiences—all while avoiding the pitfalls and numbing side effects of current medications—then its "magic" honorific is well-earned.

Psilocybin may also help combat drug addiction. In a study conducted at Johns Hopkins University in 2014, researchers found that psilocybin helped longtime cigarette smokers kick their habit. When smokers were given two to three doses of psilocybin in conjunction with cognitive-behavioral therapy, 80 percent quit smoking—and remained tobacco free for more than six months. The best available treatments today claim only a 35 percent success rate. A similar study showed that for alcoholics receiving "motivational enhancement therapy" to help them quit drinking, a dose or two of psilocybin greatly improved success rates for up to nine months.

In a 2017 study that examined survey responses from nearly half a million people, researchers found that past psychedelic use was linked to a lower incidence of criminal offenses. People who had ever used a psychedelic, including LSD and psilocybin, were 27 percent less likely to have committed larceny or theft and 22 percent less likely to have committed a violent crime in the past year. Psilocybin in particular showed a powerful beneficial effect. Use of other substances such as cocaine and heroin, however, was linked to increased likelihood of criminal offenses. Coming more than fifty years after the Concord Prison Experiment, the results seem to reaffirm Timothy Leary's hypothesis that psilocybin reduces criminal behavior. Perhaps someday we will see innovative criminal rehabilitation programs that incorporate psychedelic therapy, just as Leary's graduate students did half a century ago.

Finally, psilocybin and other psychedelics may hold the key to treating a debilitating condition known as cluster headaches. According to many who have tried the illicit substances, cluster headaches are stopped in their tracks by a dose of magic mushrooms. Perhaps, in the future, psilocybin or another psychedelic will emerge as a mainstream medicine for the many who suffer from cluster headaches.

A RECONCILIATION OF SCIENCE AND SPIRITUALITY?

From ecstasy to enlightenment, samadhi to satori, mystical states of consciousness have been known by many names in many cultures. They're highly sought after by monks, prophets, gurus, yogis, and other seekers, yet they remain notoriously elusive. As a result, mystical states have been something of a thorn in the side of psychology for many years, even as they remain the basis and highest goal of many religions.

Yet with studies like those conducted by Walter Pahnke and Roland Griffiths, science has confirmed what shamans and seers have known for millennia—that psychedelics serve as reliable portals to the most revered states of consciousness. If this research doesn't demonstrate that religion and science can indeed work harmoniously together, bearing fruit for skeptics and sages alike, nothing can.

In five hundred years, society has made little progress in the handling of sacred fungi: The attitude of today's politicians and drug enforcement agencies remains as fanatically dedicated to suppressing the mushrooms as the Conquistadors half a millennium earlier.

But empires rise and empires fall. The humble mushroom, custodian of the bridge that leads to esoteric realms of consciousness, remains impervious. María Sabina's "little children" continue to spring up wherever conditions are right, and the ranks of the age-old mushroom cult continue to grow—with or without the approval of the authorities.

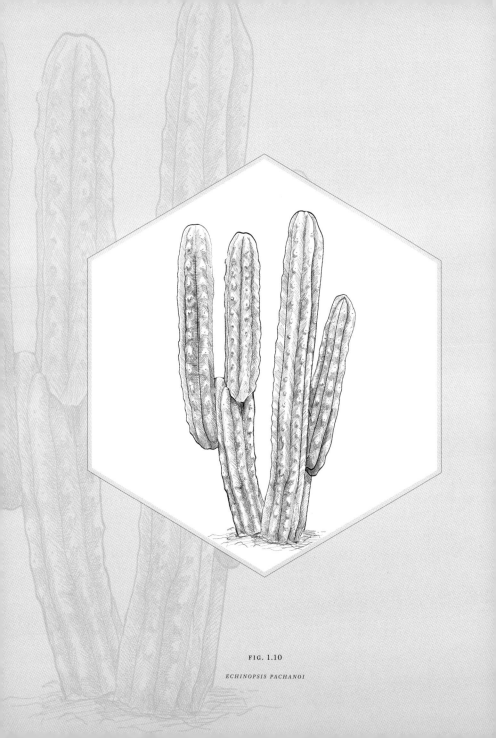

FIG. 1.10

ECHINOPSIS PACHANOI

DISCOVERED

Used by indigenous
peoples for more than
three thousand years

SAN PEDRO

ASSOCIATED WITH *indigenous peoples in Peru, Bolivia, Ecuador, Argentina, and Chile*

KEY COMPOUND *mescaline*

ORIGINS AND BACKGROUND

THOUGH IT GROWS IN THE SUN, SAN PEDRO has been thriving in the shade of relative obscurity for many decades. In popular culture, the cactus is overshadowed by Peru's much better known entheogen, ayahuasca (see page 35), whose popularity has erupted in recent decades. Today, ayahuasca is a cottage industry that draws thousands of spiritual tourists to the jungle every year, but very few make the trek for the equally powerful San Pedro ceremonies.

And as a mescaline-containing plant, San Pedro is outshined by its cousin the peyote cactus, whose ceremonial use has expanded from the Chihua-huan Desert of Mexico to various Native American tribes across the United States. Though they produce the same psychedelic compound, peyote and San Pedro cacti thrive in very different habitats on separate continents and have unique traditions of use among the indigenous tribes that revere them.

San Pedro's relative obscurity is no fault of the plant itself, which is prevalent throughout the Andes Mountains of South America. Unlike peyote, which takes decades to mature into a short, inconspicuous button, the San Pedro is a tall, fast-growing giant. Its stalks can easily grow to 10 or 20 feet (3 to 6 m) in height, and a plant often grows 12 inches (30.5 cm) or more in a year.

San Pedro has been in continuous use in South America for at least three millennia. As an indicator of its influence and staying power, images of San Pedro cacti appear—alongside deer, hummingbirds, and jaguars, as well as swirling motifs associated with its visionary effects—on ceramic artifacts sourced from distinct Andean cultures living in different centuries.

It must have been highly regarded by the Chavín people, a pre-Incan civilization in Peru, because they decorated their clothing, pottery, and holy places with its distinctive form. In a temple high in the mountains of northern Peru, archaeologists found a stone carving depicting a god holding the cactus. That carving dates to around 1300 BCE, but there is older evidence yet: At another Chavín site, the Peruvian archeologist Rosa Fung discovered remnants of what appear to be cigarlike tubes of rolled San Pedro flesh. These remains dated to 2200 BCE—more than two millennia before Saint Peter, the plant's namesake, walked the earth.

The spirit of San Pedro—or achuma, as it is often called by the natives—has been sought for many purposes through the centuries. Chief among these are diagnosing and treating various illnesses, strengthening familial and tribal bonds, and purifying the body and spirit. As a powerful spiritual medicine, it is employed not only to cure mental illnesses, such as insanity, depression, and alcoholism, but also to combat witchcraft and curses.

Such noble concerns are not always necessary, however—San Pedro may also be used simply to improve one's luck or to locate a lost item. The natives believe the cactus bears knowledge and that a person consuming its juices will encounter the answers to the questions in his heart. It is even said to foretell the future.

THE SAN PEDRO CEREMONY IN THE MODERN AGE

The San Pedro ritual is alive and well today. Tall stacks of the cacti are displayed in village markets, their thick green stalks cast alongside more prosaic fruits and vegetables. In such a setting, one could easily pass them by like so many cucumbers. But ordinary looks belie extraordinary powers. If you partake of the sacramental tea made from their flesh, all doubt vanishes: These plants offer passage to a realm that's anything but normal.

Modern shamans prepare the cactus the same way their ancestors did. The stalk is first sliced into cross sections and boiled for hours into a concentrated brew, which is then strained and drunk cold. Other psychoactive "plant teachers" are often added to this potion, including tobacco, coca leaves, *Brugmansia*—a daturalike tree in the nightshade family—and vilca, a tree whose seedpods teem with the unusual compound bufotenine. Occasionally, powdered bones or cemetery dust is added to the brew to heighten its potency further.

The final potion is called *cimora* and always served at night. To prepare, the faithful gather together to pray and invoke the powers above—both Christian saints and the spirits honored since pre-Hispanic time. The shaman holds space for his people, directing energies by blowing tobacco smoke, shaking his ceremonial rattle in a deliberate rhythm, and leading the sacred chants. At the stroke of midnight, the potion is passed around, and everyone imbibes.

THE EXPERIENCE

Like its cousin peyote, San Pedro is a dyed-in-the-wool psychedelic plant. The 8- to 12-hour trip usually includes all the mind-blowing hallmarks of psychedelia: kaleidoscopic visions, profound epiphanies, intense or even contradictory feelings, and distortions of time and space, for starters. Though the visual hallucinations can be astounding in their own right, they often take a backseat to the spiritual and emotional qualities of the experience. A bit of nausea is common, but usually subsides.

As with the other visionary plants they encountered, the Catholic Spaniards who colonized Peru condemned San Pedro. "This is the plant," wrote one missionary,

with which the devil deceived the Indians . . . in their paganism, using it for their lies and superstitions . . . those who drink lose consciousness and remain as if dead.

. . . Transported by the drink, the Indians dreamed a thousand absurdities and believed them as if they were true . . .

Reluctantly, the missionary acknowledged the medicinal qualities of the cactus, which he claimed cured fevers, hepatitis, and "burning in the bladder." The words of a Peruvian shaman, relayed by ethnobotanist Christian Rätsch, are more illuminating. At first, San Pedro produces

drowsiness or a dreamy state and a feeling of lethargy . . . a slight dizziness . . . then a great "vision," a clearing of all the faculties. . . . It produces a light numbness in the body and afterward a tranquility. And then comes detachment, a type of visual force . . . inclusive of all the senses . . . including the sixth sense, the telepathic sense of transmitting oneself across time and matter . . . like a kind of removal of one's thought to a distant dimension.

A modern user describes the effect of San Pedro as a powerful, meditative trance: "There was no difference between the inside and the outside," writes Philip Cooper, "no boundaries between the mountain and me. . . . I felt I was experiencing my true nature with everything around me. My consciousness was taking everything in on an elemental, prelingual basis. There was no distraction."

Before taking the cactus, Cooper adds, "transcendental states were just hearsay or only accessible through so much meditation and hard work. On the San Pedro, I was suddenly there."

CATHOLIC SPAIN AND THE ANCESTORS OF THE ANDES

The missionaries may not have succeeded in suppressing San Pedro ceremonies the way they did with peyote and "magic" psilocybin mushrooms, but they did transform its use. Today's curanderos, or healers, perform such heavily Christianized rituals it's difficult to determine what a precolonial ceremony might have looked like. Even San Pedro's name—a nod to Saint Peter—reflects the influence of the Spanish missionaries. How exactly the cactus came upon its saintly moniker remains a mystery, but some say it's because both Saint Peter and his spiny namesake bear keys to the kingdom of heaven.

The "mesa"—a ceremonial table prepared with sacred objects to help direct a San Pedro session—offers a striking demonstration of the modern ritual's syncretic nature: A Virgin Mary statue and a vessel of holy water may stand next to charms, seashells, and ancestral artifacts while the shaman prays to spirit guardians in thick Peruvian Spanish. It's a spiritual practice like no other in the world, a product of the region's unique history: of conquistadors and spilled blood, yes, but also of healing and deep reverence for nature.

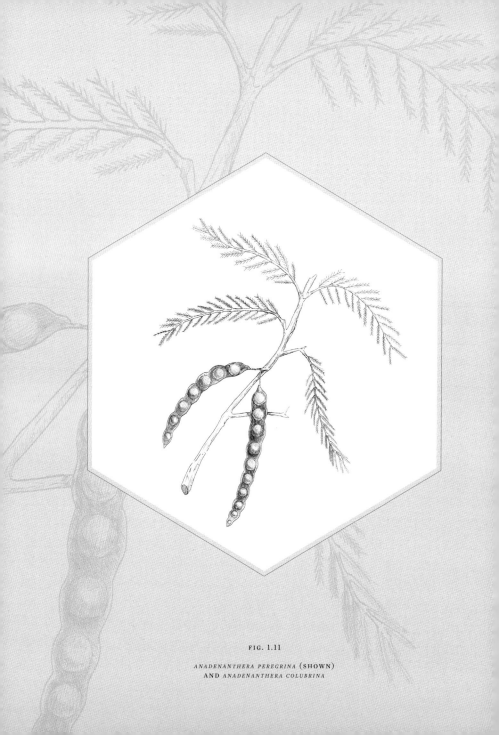

FIG. 1.11

ANADENANTHERA PEREGRINA (SHOWN)
AND *ANADENANTHERA COLUBRINA*

YOPO AND
VILCA BEANS

ASSOCIATED WITH *various South American peoples*

KEY COMPOUND *bufotenine*

ORIGINS AND BACKGROUND

Though little known among psychedelic enthusiasts of modern Western cultures, the seeds of *Anadenanthera* trees—variously known as yopo, cohoba, cebil, or vilca—have long garnered great respect among indigenous cultures in South America. In parts of Colombia, Peru, Brazil, Venezuela, and Argentina, shamans use these seeds as everything from healing medicines and divination tools to casual stimulants and even hunting aids. At one time, the use of *Anadenanthera* snuffs also spread across much of the Caribbean.

When Spanish invaders first observed yopo ceremonies in the fifteenth century, they were horrified. As zealous Catholics with no visionary sacraments of their own, they could only conclude the natives were possessed by demons. After taking yopo and tobacco, wrote one missionary in 1560, the natives, "become drowsy while the devil, in their dreams, shows them all the vanities and corruptions he wishes them to say and which they take to be true revelations."

The natives didn't see it that way. To many tribes, especially in the Orinoco River basin of Colombia and Venezuela, these seeds served—and continue to serve—vital spiritual and medicinal functions. Shamans would inhale the powder to learn the nature of a patient's disease and combat it, or to protect his tribe from witchcraft and illness, or to foretell the future. Among some tribes, yopo also served a more casual function, being used by adult males as a stimulant or consciousness enhancer.

Anadenanthera species are tall, hardy trees, growing to 60 feet (18 m) in height, with narrow branches and small round leaves that resemble those of locusts. They are immediately identifiable by the footlong (30.5 cm) seedpods dangling from their branches, which bear between six and sixteen seeds of a brilliant blood red hue. To unlock the tree's powers, the natives remove the seeds, roast them over a fire, grind them to a fine powder, and forcefully inhale them through their nostrils.

ORACLE OF THE ORINOCO

The hub of yopo's cultural influence is the basin of the Orinoco River, which defines the border between Colombia and Venezuela. The native terms "yopo" and "cohoba" refer specifically to *Anadenanthera peregrina*. A similar species—*A. colubrina*—grows in Peru and Argentina, where it is known as vilca or cebil. The proliferation of different names gives some indication of the great diversity of preparations and intentions for these remarkable seeds.

Richard Spruce, a nineteenth-century naturalist who wrote extensively about the native use of cohoba, noted that one Brazilian tribe would take the snuff before a hunt to heighten their focus. Another report from 1741 even claims that yopo was taken to prepare warriors for warfare: "Before a battle, they would throw themselves into a frenzy with Yupa, wound themselves and, full of blood and rage, go forth to battle like rabid jaguars."

The use of these seeds probably predates the Spanish conquest by many centuries. Hundreds of snuff trays and other paraphernalia have been revealed in archeological digs throughout much of South America, indicating a long and constant relationship between man and these seeds. The oldest evidence comes from northwestern Argentina, where many ceramic pipes have been discovered—some with the remains of cebil seeds inside them—which date back almost five millennia. This region boasts the longest uninterrupted ritualistic shamanic use of any psychoactive substance in the world.

Native traditions allow for many ways to consume yopo and vilca. The seeds may be eaten, which is said to cause intense vomiting, or simply chewed and held in the mouth until the active compounds are absorbed through the mucous membranes. A few tribes smoke the seeds, which produces a shorter, more intense experience. Among some cultures, the leaves and seeds are even crushed into a liquid and used for enemas. According to at least one modern scholar, the plants are indeed psychoactive when absorbed rectally—oh, the glamour of studying indigenous intoxicants.

Most often, however, the seeds are roasted, pulverized into a snuff, and inhaled into the nostrils, usually with the aid of honored artifacts, including polished wooden snuff trays and strawlike tubes made of heron bones. Often, but not always, the powder is mixed with lime from snail shells or the ashes of other plants before snuffing.

Inhaling the snuff produces an intense burning sensation and a fit of sneezing. As the active compound begins to take hold, the shaman will shiver, convulse, and enter a state of frenzied delirium. It's no wonder early Spaniards saw the work of the devil as they observed the fire-lit faces of natives contorting into

COHOBA, THE CARIBBEAN SNUFF

There is evidence that yopo snuffs were once cultivated and consumed throughout the Caribbean. Snuffing artifacts from preconquest times have been discovered throughout the Greater Antilles. Christopher Columbus, on his second voyage to the New World, remarked upon the Taíno natives on the island of Hispaniola, who would sniff a powder and "lose consciousness and become like drunken men."

A friar hired by Columbus to study the Taíno culture wrote that this intoxicating snuff was called cohoba. "They take it with a cane about a foot long [30.5 cm]," wrote the friar, "and put one end in the nose and the other in the powder" to inhale the snuff. Yet, the botanical source of this snuff remained an enduring mystery. More than four hundred years later, cohoba was finally identified as *Anadenanthera peregrina*—the same plant as yopo.

grotesque positions, shrieking with wild eyes and running noses, after sniffing the "malignant powder."

After this initial phase, the shaman begins speaking in tongues and gesticulating wildly, a language of the whole body understood only by the spirits. If he is treating a sick patient, the shaman learns from the spirits the nature of the illness and draws on their powers to cure it.

As is typical of psychedelics, the inner experience is more illuminating than the physical effects apparent to bystanders. The visions last for 20 minutes, and, according to some sources, usually appear in black and white. The hallucinations, in contrast to many other psychedelics, tend toward flowing arabesque shapes rather than linear, geometric patterns. It is rare for the visions to take any realistic or figurative forms, instead remaining abstract. At high doses and in low light, these swirling motifs may surround the user in three dimensions, eminently real yet untouchable.

Perhaps unsurprisingly, this painful habit of sniffing these powders has not caught on outside of its native context. Nor has bufotenine, the chief psychoactive component, emerged as a desirable compound on the modern recreational market, the way other native intoxicants have, such as cocaine, mescaline, and DMT. In fact, hardly anyone cops to having consumed pure bufotenine, and those who have rarely recommend the experience.

BUFOTENINE: THE SECRET OF YOPO?

There has been much debate about bufotenine, the major alkaloid in the seeds of the *Anadenanthera* species. First, there is the question of whether it is psychoactive at all, which was doubted for many years, and also whether it is truly responsible for the visionary effects of yopo and vilca snuffs. The snuffs also contain DMT and 5-MeO-DMT (see pages 45 and 29)—powerful psychedelic compounds in their own right—but their concentrations are negligible compared to that of bufotenine. Structurally, bufotenine is closely related to DMT, psilocin—the "magic" in magic mushrooms (see page 89)— and one of the brain's chief chemical messengers, serotonin. Yet unlike these chemical cousins, bufotenine's nature remains contentious.

Early studies, marred by questionable ethical standards, characterized pure bufotenine as a toxin rather than a psychedelic. Scientists who injected the substance to schizophrenic patients and convicts observed alarming results, including extreme salivation, burning sensations, and faces so flushed they turned purple. The scientists were forced to stop their research, and bufotenine was quickly slated for Schedule I, the most prohibitive drug classification in the United States.

More recent studies have shown an unexpected result—people with schizophrenia and autism have significant concentrations of natural bufotenine in their urine. Scientists speculate the compound may play a role in these conditions, though whether it's a cause or a byproduct remains unclear.

Not limited to the plant kingdom, bufotenine also appears in the venom of a family of toads—the genus *Bufo*, from which the compound derives its unusual name. This has led to the oft-publicized but rarely encountered phenomenon of "toad licking"—a dangerous pastime, as these frogs' venom contain a dizzying variety of "bufotoxins" so dangerous they make bufotenine look like chamomile tea (see pages 29 and 30).

After trying the drug, ethnobotanist Jonathan Ott described one recurring characteristic, a "shimmery 'magical varnish' (to borrow Baudelaire's bon mot) over the world, which seems to breathe." At other times he experienced, "a sudden and dramatic dimming of the visual field, as though the starting of a heavy motor had dropped line-voltage and dimmed the lights." He felt one thing for certain: Pure bufotenine was indeed psychoactive. Though he remarked on its unique and idiosyncratic effects, Ott, like most psychonauts dedicated enough to try this compound, did not enjoy the experience.

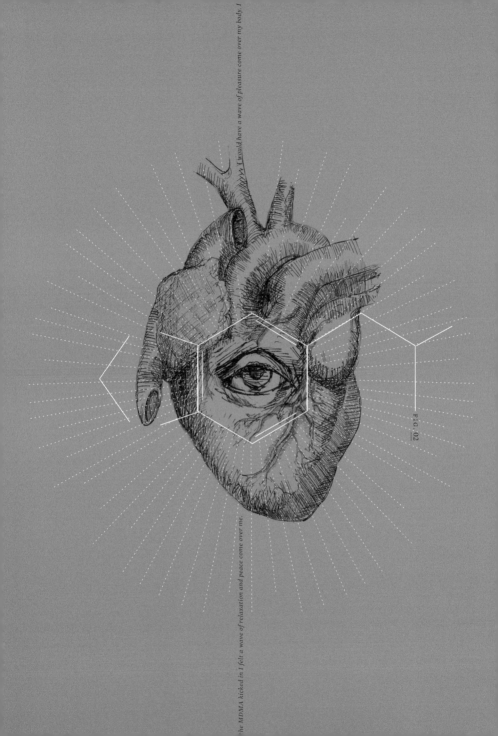

As the MDMA kicked in I felt a wave of relaxation and peace come over me. I would have a wave of pleasure come over my body. I

FIG. 02

CHAPTER TWO

EMPATHOGENIC PSYCHEDELICS

Though less overtly "trippy" than other substances, the empathogens —literally "creating empathy"—still amplify emotions and insights in a decidedly psychedelic way. The crown jewel of the empathogens is MDMA—better known as Ecstasy—which today leads the revival of psychedelic medicine.

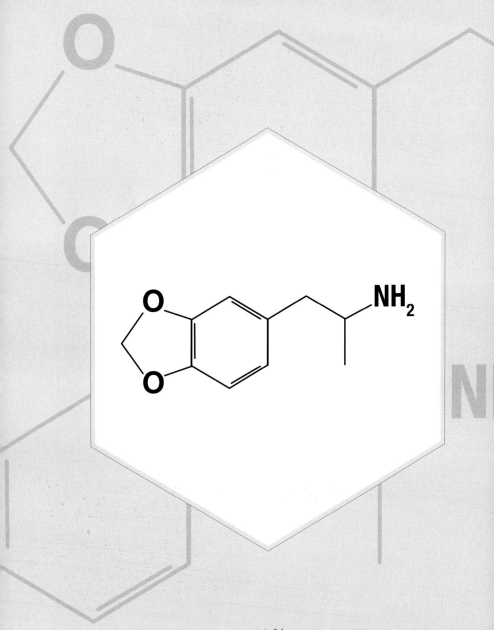

FIG. 2.1

3,4-METHYLENEDIOXYAMPHETAMINE

DISCOVERED		DURATION
German chemists Carl Mannich and Willy Jacobsohn in 1910	**MDA**	4 to 6 hours

ASSOCIATED WITH *psychedelic 1960s and experimental psychotherapy*

ORIGINS AND BACKGROUND

THOUGH LITTLE KNOWN TODAY, MDA WAS THE ORIGINAL "love drug." A popular and widely available substance in the 1960s and '70s, MDA was renowned among both psychedelic enthusiasts and therapists for its euphoric, empathetic, and sometimes even spiritual effects.

MDA made a splash as the first true empathogen—a substance engendering feelings of closeness, openness, and trust—almost twenty years before its chemical cousin MDMA caused a worldwide sensation under the name of Ecstasy. In the pre-Ecstasy era, MDA's enhancement of emotional openness was both highly desirable and utterly unique. And as the compound lacked the tongue-tying and often bewildering effects of stronger psychedelics such as LSD, it was more suitable to social and therapeutic situations.

MDA was first developed by German chemists at the pharmaceutical company Merck in 1910, just two years before scientists at the same lab discovered MDMA. It was examined at various times as a potential cough suppressant, diet aid, and antidepressant, but it never became a prescription medicine. Even the U. S. Army took an interest, testing the drug as a possible truth serum or brainwashing agent in a series of illegal—and ill-fated—experiments in the 1950s (see page 66).

MDA really came into its own in the early '60s, when free-loving hippies and forward-thinking therapists got wind of its profound emotional effects. But like LSD, psilocybin, and all other substances associated with the era's countercultural movement, MDA was swiftly banned. Once a promising therapeutic agent in the same vein as MDMA, MDA research has dwindled to virtually zero.

GORDON ALLES'S MAIDEN VOYAGE

For every molecular concoction, some brave soul must serve as the first explorer. Gordon Alles, a pharmacologist who had discovered amphetamine in 1927, took that plunge when he became the first person to ingest MDA in 1930.

The physical symptoms came on first: tension in the neck and jaw, a compulsion to grind his teeth, and huge, dilated pupils. Alles recognized these signs from his experience with two other stimulants—amphetamine and ephedrine. That's when he noticed the smoke rings. Alles knew there was no smoke in the lab, and yet he perceived, "an abundance of curling smoke rings," utterly convincing in the way they wafted about. Yet ,when he passed a finger through them, "they melted away."

Paradoxically, Alles also reported improved visual acuity. He was seeing things that weren't there, yes, but the things that *were* there, he perceived with eagle-eyed clarity. Looking out the window, he found he could observe faraway scenes in "very minute detail."

Then, things took a strange turn. In a relaxed state, Alles found himself drifting out of his body and into "a detached place of observation," floating in the air like one of the ghostly smoke rings he'd just encountered. As the scientist watched, his center of consciousness was

transposed out of the body and to a place above and to the right rearward.
I was compelled to turn my head several times and look into that upper corner of
the room in wonder at what part of me could be up there . . .

Then, he began hearing footsteps. Peeking his head out of the room, he found no one in the corridor. Yet the footsteps persisted. Finally, he looked out his sixth-floor window. Sure enough, every time he heard footsteps, he saw a

MAGIC MEDICINE

| 118 |

pedestrian walking down the sidewalk far below. The researcher was astounded—the distant shuffling of feet, too soft to have ever warranted his attention before, now resonated with crystal clarity and commanded his full concentration.

THE EXPERIENCE

MDA defies easy categorization. Because of its tendency to produce emotional warmth and openness, it is often classed as an empathogen (generating empathy) alongside MDMA. But compared to MDMA, MDA is more stimulating, providing a "rush" like that of cocaine or amphetamine. It sometimes exhibits trippy qualities, such as synesthesia (blending of the senses), slowing of time, and an ineffable sense of oneness with the universe, but these pale in comparison to stronger psychedelics. Milder than LSD yet more mind-bending than amphetamine, MDA occupies an agreeable middle ground somewhere between stimulants, psychedelics, and empathogens.

For most people, MDA is not an especially visual molecule; the most prominent effects are emotional. A small 1974 study summarized the effects nicely: Most of the subjects felt, "more relaxed, happier and more at peace with the world during the experience," as well as "more calm, more free, more loving and felt more like paying close attention to their surroundings." Even more striking, more than half the subjects reported

> that as a result of the experience, the meaning of life was clearer, that life has new significance and that they were able to discern new connections between certain events or experiences that they had not been aware of before.

With its ability to break through people's internal barriers, the researchers speculated MDA may offer help to those struggling with "obsessive, anxious, or depressive patterns" of thinking. They found the substance facilitated "increased introspectiveness, heightened self-awareness, and greater intuitiveness [as well as] relaxation, acceptance, calmness and serenity"—the perfect mix of qualities for psychotherapy.

MDA research lay dormant for more than thirty years, but in 2010, Matthew Baggott led a study showing MDA induces "mystical" experiences. These powerful states, known throughout history to prophets, mystics, and gurus of all religions, are characterized by a sense of oceanic boundlessness, transcendence of normal reality, and oneness with all things.

William James, the father of American psychology, described the mystical state as the "root and center" of all religious experience. Psychedelics have long been associated with transcendent experiences, but this research confirms that empathogens, too, can act as doorways to the divine. With the right molecular portal, this once-rarefied state of consciousness—regarded by some as the pinnacle moments of their lives—is available to everyone.

Of course, not everyone is interested in MDA's therapeutic or spiritual effects. As with Ecstasy, it has also been used at parties, dance clubs, and music festivals by people attracted to its euphoric and empathic qualities. Whether on the dance floor or a therapist's couch, MDA promotes self-acceptance and uninhibited expression. For the recreationally minded, the boundless energy doesn't hurt either.

SIDE EFFECTS

Though a relatively safe substance when taken under medical supervision, MDA has its share of dangers. As a strong stimulant, it can be dangerous for people with heart conditions or high blood pressure. But an overdose can be life threatening for anyone, and a few fatalities have been reported (see sidebar MDA and Secret Experiments, page 121).

Given MDA's prevalence of use, the overall incidence of medical emergencies is quite low. For most users, the main concerns are psychological, as the substance can surface unwanted memories or feelings and lead to overwhelming sensations.

The most extensive MDA studies were conducted by Norman Zinberg at Harvard Medical School and published in 1976. Zinberg characterized its main effect on perception as "a de-automatization of repetitive, usual modes of responding" to the world, allowing subjects to apply their full focus to very specific details of their environment. This narrowing of concentration—or rather, the expansion of an individual detail to occupy one's entire consciousness—struck Zinberg as one of MDA's most powerful effects.

Zinberg also reported on the compound's remarkable enhancement of empathy. He found that people on MDA paid such close attention to the subtle cues of those around them that they were able to perform apparent acts of mind reading.

Not only was such a subject able to describe what others felt, e.g., "A is thinking of sex with B," or, "I think C is lost in childhood memories or relationship fantasies with D," but they were also able to say something about the cues that led to these conclusions—the way someone's body was now dripping with sand, the way the lines formed around a person's mouth, or the way somebody looked over there and then looked away.

MDA AND SECRET EXPERIMENTS

In 1952, a forty-two-year old tennis player named Harold Blauer checked himself into the New York State Psychiatric Institute complaining of severe depression in the wake of a divorce. Unbeknownst to Blauer, the hospital had a secret agreement with the U.S. Army to administer experimental drugs to patients, as part of the MKUltra project, in which thousands of unsuspecting victims were dosed without their knowledge or consent (see page 66).

Blauer died after receiving an intravenous injection of 450 milligrams of MDA—a strong dose many times over. His medical records were modified to exonerate the hospital, and the truth about his death only came out twenty-two years later, when Blauer's family won a settlement of more than $700,000.

Most of the time, these assertions turned out to be correct. "It was remarkable," Zinberg wrote, "and it gave me some sense of why some psychedelic users of my acquaintance had become so interested in ESP."

THE FORGOTTEN PSYCHEDELIC THERAPY

MDMA-assisted therapy gets all the press these days, thanks to major studies examining its potential as a treatment for post-traumatic stress disorder (PTSD), but MDA once claimed a leading role in psychotherapy. Before its prohibition in 1970, MDA gained traction as a unique and powerful therapeutic tool. Crucially, it improved rapport between therapist and client—the cornerstone of any talk therapy approach—but that was just the beginning.

MDA quelled patients' fears and anxieties, and it allowed people to revisit painful memories without feeling threatened or overwhelmed. In a state of serenity and self-acceptance, patients reported increased self-insight, greater understanding of their relationships, and an attitude of forgiveness for their own mistakes. With the ego out of the way, epiphanies became the norm. For patients whose attempts at healing had been thwarted by their own self-defense mechanisms, MDA was just what the doctor ordered.

Two influential figures were Leo Zeff, a psychologist and leader in the psychedelic therapy movement, and Claudio Naranjo, a Chilean psychiatrist with groundbreaking ideas about integrating therapy, spirituality, and substances he called "emotion-enhancers." Both used MDA extensively in their personal therapy practices and spoke candidly about its value in inducing cathartic and insightful sessions.

Zeff valued its ability to reorient people to the current moment, eliminating distractions from the past and speculations about the future.

MDA clarifies your life, puts everything in a correct perspective for you . . .
You come out with a good feeling about yourself. It helps you to see all your
difficulties in a different light, and they cease to be difficulties. . . .
It brings you into the experience of the moment.

For Naranjo, MDA's chief value lay in its powerful ability to retrieve old memories. Regression to childhood "occurs so frequently and spontaneously that this can be considered a typical effect of this substance, and a prime source of its therapeutic value." According to Naranjo, episodes of "age regression" play a critical role in a person's journey of healing.

Such trials require significant funds and the navigation of complex bureaucratic hurdles, however, so while MDMA marches ever closer to prescription status, legalized MDA-assisted therapy remains a distant dream. It's a cruel irony that the original love drug—so magnetic and memorable in its effects— should be left behind and forgotten, buried in the sands of history without so much as a good-bye.

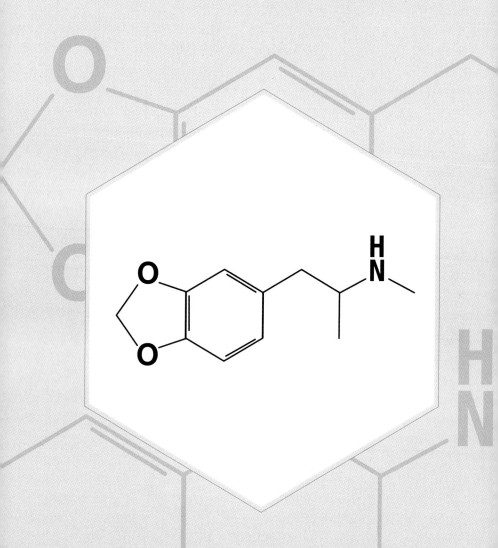

FIG. 2.2

3,4-METHYLENEDIOXYMETHAMPHETAMINE

ALSO KNOWN AS *Ecstasy, Molly, X*

ASSOCIATED WITH *raves and electronic dance music; psychotherapy for PTSD*

ORIGINS AND BACKGROUND

M DMA RANKS AS ONE OF THE MOST INFLUENTIAL and famous—or infamous—pharmacological discoveries of the twentieth century. Its rise and fall, from an experimental therapy to demonized social menace, mirrored that of LSD a generation earlier. Compared to the psychedelics of the '60s, however, MDMA offered gentler, more reliable effects, earning it a wide appeal among those who wanted an altered state without hallucinations or the risk of a "bad trip."

From raves and music festivals to therapists' offices and couples' bedrooms, in bars and nightclubs and homes around the world, tens of millions of people have enjoyed its charms. Almost 7 percent of American adults—more than twenty million people—have tried MDMA in their lives.

Its unique ability to break down psychic dams, releasing torrents of emotion in a manageable, nonthreatening way, earned MDMA a reputation as a miracle drug among adventurous psychiatrists and patients. Though first created in 1912, its astounding emotional effects did not come to light until the 1970s, when it spread across a worldwide network of unorthodox therapists who appreciated its "heart-opening" quality.

Before long, though, the "love drug"—commonly known as "Ecstasy"—escaped into the recreational market and became a staple of the 1980s dance and club scene. True to its name, Ecstasy's euphoric and empathogenic qualities found a receptive audience among ravers and clubbers, who used it not only to improve their stamina on the dance floor but to engender a powerful sense of connection with every person they encountered.

Even as Ecstasy exploded in popularity, its advocates in the mental health community remained hopeful about its potential to revolutionize the therapeutic process. They were disappointed: Though MDMA was well tolerated under controlled conditions, its effects "in the wild" were less predictable, and a spate of deaths and hospitalizations led to a worldwide crackdown in the mid-1980s. Just like that, the promising avenue of MDMA research reached a dead end.

Today, MDMA research is flourishing once again, thanks to the pioneering nonprofit organization MAPS. Led by longtime MDMA and psychedelic research advocate Rick Doblin, MAPS is developing the compound as a prescription medicine for people struggling with the aftereffects of trauma. In a few years, MDMA's journey may come full circle: from promising medicine to dance club bombshell to black market drug and finally to accepted medicine.

THE EXPERIENCE

It's easy to see why MDMA appeals to such a diverse cross section of society. If alcohol is a social lubricant, MDMA is a full tune-up of body and mind, generating a sense of physical, emotional, and spiritual well-being. It temporarily smoothes over the cracks of doubt and despair that mar even the hardiest of human souls. For a few hours, it paints a picture of true mental health, insecurities crowded out by bubbles of confidence and an all-encompassing sense of serenity. Far from an escape, it feels more like a coming to terms—with oneself, with reality, with the blessed beauty of existence. Enthusiasts say it can provide all the personal insights of psilocybin or LSD, without the mind-bending and, sometimes, dark surprises these psychedelics are known for.

As an agent of openness, MDMA allows uninhibited communication of difficult or repressed subjects among friends, lovers, and therapists and their clients. As a stimulant, it intensifies one's focus and attention to razorlike sharpness, while unleashing reservoirs of latent energy. And in an age of distraction, MDMA demands engagement—with the immediate environment, with the needs and desires of people nearby, with one's own body, and with fears and insecurities long suppressed. In its uncanny ability to engender a sense of serenity and self-acceptance, MDMA is unmatched.

Physical effects are similar to other amphetamine-based stimulants: seemingly endless energy, muscle tension, teeth grinding, and pupils wide as saucers. MDMA also enhances the pleasure from exercise and tactile sensations—dance, touch, and massage transcend the realm of merely "pleasant" activities and become sublime, even for those normally too shy to partake. Sex is another story—though erotic touch is amplified, many men find it very difficult to achieve an erection. The paradox of the "love drug" is that it unites minds and bodies together, but stymies efforts at sexual communion.

THE GODFATHER OF ECSTASY AND THE PSYCHEDELIC THERAPIST

It's incredible that researchers discovering MDMA's unique effects would be anything but, well, ecstatic. Yet, after Merck patented it back in 1912, the substance mostly languished in obscurity for half a century. The U. S. Army thought it was worth a look, conducting classified research of its toxicity and behavioral effects in animals in the early 1950s, but they, too, failed to yield any substantial results. In fact, were it not for the efforts of two men who believed in its power to transform the human psyche for the better, MDMA would likely remain a forgotten substance today.

Alexander Shulgin first popularized MDMA among therapists—indirectly leading to its immense popularity as a recreational drug. After a student turned him on to the little-known drug in 1976, Shulgin introduced it to Leo Zeff, a psychologist who had developed groundbreaking methods for incorporating substances such as LSD and MDA into his therapy practice. MDMA quickly earned a place in his therapeutic toolbox.

In fact, Zeff was so taken with the MDMA experience he postponed his retirement, traveling around the United States and Europe to train thousands of other psychologists in MDMA-assisted psychotherapy. It quickly gained a reputation among therapists as an impressive catalyst for emotional openness, with patients

If alcohol is a social lubricant, MDMA is a full tune-up of body and mind, generating a sense of physical, emotional, and spiritual well-being.

often showing more progress in a single session than in years of traditional talk therapy.

THE BIRTH OF THE RAVE

In the 1980s, Ecstasy exploded into mainstream usage. As yuppies, psychedelic users, and students began taking it in earnest, a distribution network sprang up in Texas to meet the demand—complete with a pyramid sales structure and toll-free phone numbers where credit cards were gladly accepted. The distributors coined the name "Ecstasy" to enhance its allure and increase sales, advertising it as a "fun drug" that was "good to dance to."

Customers agreed. Soon, "Ecstasy parties" became the new trend at many bars, nightclubs, and colleges around the country, and the Texas entrepreneurs were selling as many as two hundred thousand tablets a month. At one time, you could actually walk into bars in Dallas and Austin and buy Ecstasy over the counter. When Texans advertised happy hour, they meant it.

In England, MDMA became the go-to substance at "acid house" parties—unlicensed events held in large warehouses, featuring heavy bass music. The years 1988 and 1989 were dubbed the Second Summer of Love due to the simultaneous explosion of electronic dance music, huge hedonistic parties, and copious amounts of MDMA. From these humble roots grew the rave scene—today an international phenomenon with its own values, fashions, dance moves, and accessories.

Early raves were unauthorized events, often held at abandoned industrial warehouses or in suburban countryside meadows. Locations were communicated at the last minute to avoid interference from the police. A typical rave featured DJs spinning house, trance, or techno tracks through a powerful sound system, while laser light shows played across synthetic fog. Especially in the United States, ravers began sporting illuminated gloves, glow sticks, and neon clothes that fluoresce under the venue's ultraviolet lights. Raves were based on the founding principles of peace, love, unity, and respect (PLUR), reminding attendees to act with kindness while raving and in their daily lives.

Today raves are bigger than ever. Having emerged from underground, the raving subculture has spawned massive festivals like Tomorrowland and Electric Daisy Carnival, which draw hundreds of thousands of attendees every year. The twenty-first century's answer to Woodstock, these festivals bring the principles and aesthetics of 1990s raves to the big stage.

With a focus on positive connections, togetherness, and love—not to mention hours of intense physical exertion—it comes as no surprise that ravers would favor MDMA over other substances.

THE CRACKDOWN

National media outlets started reporting on the MDMA sensation in 1985, often with cautious optimism as an experimental therapeutic tool. But in June of that year, the federal government banned MDMA. It was placed in the most restrictive category, Schedule I, reserved for substances with a high potential for abuse and no accepted medical use.

An outcry from psychiatrists and psychologists, who had planned to utilize MDMA's unique effects in ongoing research and therapy, culminated in a series of hearings about the substance's ultimate fate. In spite of the evidence presented at the hearings, the head of the U. S. Drug Enforcement Administration permanently confirmed MDMA's Schedule I status in 1986. This not only made criminals of all personal users but also effectively halted all research and forced MDMA psycho-therapy underground.

THE PHARMACOLOGY OF MDMA

MDMA is like that impulsive, charismatic friend whose charms you can't resist. But instead of convincing you to blow your savings on a wild weekend in Vegas, it induces the brain to release its natural stores of serotonin, dumping out happy chemicals like candy from a piñata. MDMA also acts as a potent releaser of dopamine—the chemical basis of the brain's reward network—as well as norepinephrine, a hormone that normally primes the body for action during times of emotional stress and physical activity.

MDMA also causes a spike in oxytocin, a hormone associated with social bonding, as well as cortisol, whose chief function in the body is to increase the availability of energy in the form of glucose. Both hormones may prove relevant to MDMA's role in psychotherapy: Oxytocin may strengthen the bond between therapist and patient, and cortisol could contribute to "unlearning" the fear responses that normally prevent patients from grappling with painful topics.

MDMA's method of looting the brain's pleasure treasury is also its downfall. Afterward, the brain must rebuild its stores from scratch, and many users exhibit some signs of depression, irritability, or lethargy a few days after their trip. Others, however, experience no such moody hangover, basking in the golden afterglow until their feet return to solid ground.

TOXICITY

Media reports tend to sensationalize every MDMA-related death, in stark contrast to the many deaths caused by alcohol or tobacco. In reality, MDMA has fairly low toxicity when used in moderation. Considering the millions of users who have tried it, the relatively few medical emergencies and fatalities—while unquestionably tragic—pale in comparison to other commonly accepted vices and refute MDMA's image as a toxic poison.

Used carelessly, however, MDMA can be very dangerous. Because of its dramatic effect on brain chemistry, MDMA exhibits rapid tolerance and produces withdrawal effects in regular users who quit suddenly. Dosages are not as forgiving as with psychedelics such as psilocybin mushrooms or LSD, and serious overdoses do occur. For some people, no dose is safe. In particular, because MDMA increases heart rate and blood pressure, it is not recommended for those with heart conditions. Others just react poorly, complaining of tense muscles, anxiety, and excessive sweating. Overall, though, more than 97 percent of users place a positive value on the experience afterward.

One major concern debated for decades is neurotoxicity. Early studies were conducted on animals, not humans, and with massive doses that did not correlate to typical therapeutic or recreational amounts. Nevertheless, claims of MDMA's neurotoxicity gained traction in the media and the popular consciousness and played a large role in its prohibition.

There was some truth to the claims. Later studies with humans have shown that frequent high doses of MDMA are, in fact, neurotoxic, but moderate doses do not appear to correlate with any kind of brain damage or lasting impairments. Chronic heavy users may develop structural changes to the serotonin-based neural pathways, depleted serotonin, and death and damage to neurons in key brain regions. They may show cognitive impairments and poor memory and suffer from insomnia, depression, or anxiety. The good news is, for people who use only moderate doses a few times a year, no such negative trends have been found.

In spite of what headlines may say, most deaths and medical emergencies attributed to MDMA are not overdoses. The main concerns are dehydration and heatstroke, usually as a result of dancing for hours in a hot environment without properly hydrating. MDMA can contribute to heatstroke by raising the body's temperature and interfering with normal temperature-regulation processes, but heatstroke is fairly common, even among clubbers who have not taken drugs. Education and preparatory measures, including proper air-cooling and plentiful water provided by event organizers, can help prevent this.

Several nonprofits and advocacy groups around the globe are seeking to change the approach to recreational MDMA use by focusing on "harm reduction" efforts. One method is pill testing, a service offered at progressive events such as Boom Festival in Portugal to provide attendees with real-time information about their substances. As long as MDMA remains an unregulated black market drug, pill testing will be an essential—and potentially life-saving—public health service for the millions of people who consume it.

MDMA has fairly low toxicity when used in moderation.

Although it remains a strictly controlled substance, a resurgence of interest has brought MDMA back to the forefront of psychiatry in recent years. Before its prohibition, a couple of studies provided tantalizing clues about the compound's medical potential. Participants of one study reported lasting improvements in their personal relationships, deeper insight into personal problems, and an "expanded mental perspective." Subjects also felt that "their defenses were lowered"—a key component of the therapeutic process.

Another study, conducted by a Swiss team led by Dr. Peter Gasser, examined the long-term effects of 121 patients who had undergone several MDMA-assisted therapy sessions. More than 80 percent reported enhanced quality of life, and over 90 percent experienced an improvement in the condition for which they had sought therapy. Respondents also indicated a decrease in using drugs such as alcohol and cannabis.

After its prohibition in 1985, MDMA research lay dormant for a time, but in the last decade, it has returned in full force. MAPS is now investigating MDMA-assisted therapy as a potential cure for PTSD, as well as for social anxiety in autistic adults and anxiety in people with terminal illnesses. MAPS president and founder Rick Doblin estimates that, by 2021, MDMA will be approved as a prescription treatment for PTSD in the United States. This is an ambitious goal, but MAPS has made considerable headway. In a pilot study, more than 80 percent of subjects no longer met the criteria for PTSD after their sessions—an incredible recovery rate for such a challenging and intractable condition.

Medical MDMA is groundbreaking in many ways. First, its effects are unique in the field of psychiatry—nothing even remotely similar has ever gotten so close to becoming a mainstream medicine. Most medicines prescribed for mental disorders such as PTSD and anxiety are "maintenance drugs" that must be taken every day. Usually, these treat the symptoms rather than the underlying causes, and they frequently cause unpleasant side effects while only partially resolving the condition.

In stark contrast, MDMA only needs to be taken once or twice—in the presence of specially trained therapists—to produce lasting benefits. According to researchers, that's because MDMA opens subjects up to their own "inner healing intelligence," allowing them to process traumatic memories instead of merely numbing them. MDMA-assisted therapy is a far cry from your average visit to the shrink. Not just a new medicine, MDMA offers an altogether new healing modality, where patients take the medicine in the presence of two trusted therapists in a calm and relaxing office setting.

What's the light at the end of the tunnel? The rehabilitation of MDMA as a valuable medicine and the opportunity to offer healing to the people who need it most—veterans, firefighters, police officers, victims of sexual assault, and others recovering from severe trauma. Perhaps, then, MDMA will have truly earned the title of the "love drug."

A SOLDIER'S TESTIMONIAL

In an eye-opening "Ask Me Anything" interactive session on Reddit, retired U. S. Army Sergeant Tony Macie, an Iraq War veteran, shed some light on his experience with PTSD and MDMA therapy. Like many with PTSD, his condition had failed to improve after traditional treatments such as talk therapy. Desperate for help, he enrolled in a MAPS-sponsored study, and the results were astonishing:

. . . when the MDMA kicked in I felt a wave of relaxation and peace come over me. For the first hour I did not really talk, I just laid there and enjoyed the quietness of my normally hyper vigilant mind.

. . . [That's] when memories started to come up. . . . If I tried to push them away I would feel anxious, but if I dealt with it and processed the memory, I would have a wave of pleasure come over my body. I believe that the MDMA was showing me how to deal with my trauma and also that it is more beneficial for me to face trauma head on than to try [to] ignore it or suppress it. I had a lot of powerful realizations that day.

Tony emerged a different man. No longer dogged by constant anxiety and vigilance, he quit all prescription medications and hasn't looked back.

"Instead of trying to forget experiences," he writes, "I focus on learning from them." MDMA is not a panacea, and not all PTSD sufferers will respond as positively as Tony Macie has. But he believes that if research continues to demonstrate positive results, all people with trauma deserve to have this revolutionary treatment at their disposal.

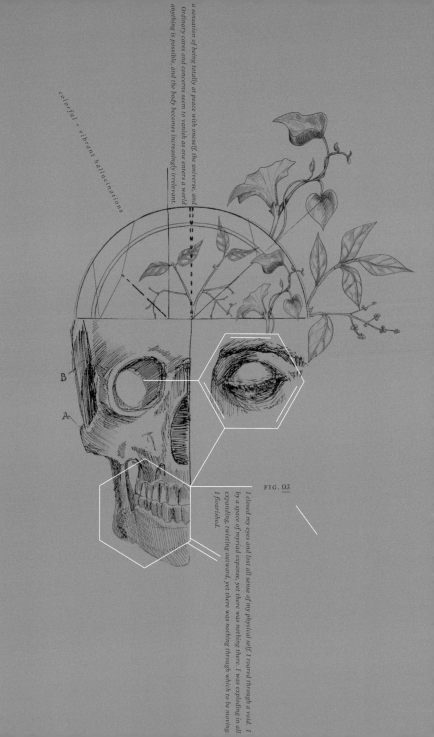

a sensation of being totally at peace with oneself; the universe, and
Ordinary cares and concerns seem to vanish as one enters a world
anything is possible, and the body becomes increasingly irrelevant.

colorful + vibrant hallucinations

B

A

FIG. 03

I closed my eyes and lost all sense of my physical self. I roared through a void. I
by a space of myriad expanse, yet there was nothing there. I was exploding in all
expanding, twisting outward, yet there was nothing through which to be moving.
I flourished.

CHAPTER THREE

DISSOCIATIVE PSYCHEDELICS

The dissociatives, so named because they distance users from their surroundings and even their own bodies, have medical uses ranging from anesthesia to cough suppression. Ketamine, the tranquilizer-cum-club-drug, is emerging as a powerful new treatment for severe depression. But beware—at higher doses, astral travel and other bizarre out-of-body experiences prevail.

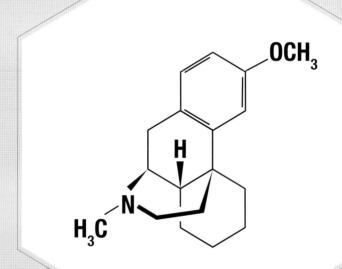

FIG. 3.1

DEXTROMETHORPHAN

DISCOVERED

Swiss chemists Andre
Grüssner and Otto Schnider
in 1946

DXM

DURATION

4 to 8 hours

BEST KNOWN AS *the main ingredient in most cough medicines*

ORIGINS AND BACKGROUND

A S AN INEXPENSIVE AND WIDELY ACCESSIBLE over-the-counter cough suppressant, dextromethorphan, or DXM, is a mainstay of household medicine cabinets everywhere. It is the only entry in this book with which almost everyone can claim some level of experience. At some point in your childhood, that cloyingly sweet syrup likely found its way past your lips. For many children, cough syrup represents the taste of medicine itself.

But as millions of teenagers—and, yes, adults—have found, DXM is good for a whole lot more than suppressing coughs. Once obscure enough to escape the notice of the medical community, DXM has emerged as the black sheep of the psychedelic family. Even recreational drug users tend to scoff at the idea of drinking cough syrup, dismissing it as the psychedelic equivalent of sniffing glue or quaffing a bottle of mouthwash—a bottom-of-the-barrel drug sought only by desperate teens who can't get ahold of the good stuff. Its shady reputation was cemented by numerous sensational headlines, warning about "millions of young people" raiding medicine cabinets for "easy-to-get" drugs.

For those willing to look, there's much more to the story. DXM's proponents point to its visionary and, arguably, shamanic powers far beyond what the headlines indicate. Our cultural attitude toward the substance stems more from ignorance and a puritanical "Just Say No" sensibility than from any qualities of the compound itself. It's natural to raise suspicion about a drug closely associated with young people, and it must be acknowledged that reckless use has resulted in a handful of avoidable deaths, but does that mean it has no value as a self-exploratory tool for cautious adults?

MORE THAN COUGH MEDICINE

Two Swiss scientists, Andre Grüssner and Otto Schnider, first discovered DXM in 1946 and patented it three years later. By the mid-1950s, the CIA and the U. S. Navy were researching DXM's potential as a nonaddictive replacement for codeine. This research fell under the auspices of MKPILOT, a secret U.S. government project that—along with another covert CIA operation, the better-known MKUltra—tested drugs for mind control or behavior modification.

In 1958, the Food and Drug Administration approved DXM as a cough suppressant, a category previously dominated by codeine. Although effective, codeine had major drawbacks—aside from causing side effects like drowsiness, it also had tremendous abuse potential and sometimes led to opioid dependence.

Of course, DXM came with its own baggage. The over-the-counter tablet formulation, Romilar, became popular as a recreational drug in its own right throughout the 1960s. Among its fans were the Beat poet Allen Ginsberg, author Jack Kerouac, and the rock critic Lester Bangs, who had this to say about dextromethorphan: "You call it a 'stone' or a 'high' because it changes your consciousness and your physical sensations. But it changes them to emptiness—a total vacuum, a total absence of self." That may not sound like a glowing endorsement, but Bangs loved the stuff and indulged frequently.

DXM AND PUNK

DXM emerged as a drug of choice in the hardcore punk scene of the 1980s. In this context, it was usually taken in group settings, and in some rural areas represented an important part of the punk subculture. Its use was by no means unanimous, however—in fact, many hardcore musicians railed against all kinds of drugs and alcohol and founded the Straight Edge movement.

In 1973, after an upswing in sales due to growing recreational usage, DXM tablets were taken off the shelves and replaced with cough syrup, a less appetizing option intended to discourage nonmedical use. For those who've wondered why cough medicine almost always comes as a syrup, the answer is simple: to make it unpleasant to consume.

The advent of the Internet in the 1990s laid the groundwork for modern DXM culture. DXM users, formerly a splintered and obscure group with only the loosest associations, were able to unite as online networks where they shared information, trip experiences, and even DXM-inspired art and music. With these online forums, the substance's popularity has increased in recent years. The secret is officially out—a powerful dissociative hallucinogen can be had for a pittance at any neighborhood drugstore.

THE EXPERIENCE

Dextromethorphan was developed as a synthetic opioid analog, but its effects are nothing like morphine and other opioids. In fact, it's more akin to dissociatives such as ketamine and PCP. At low doses, dissociatives produce euphoria, anesthesia, and unusual bodily sensations. At higher levels, they can induce profound out-of-body experiences.

Among DXM enthusiasts, the experience is often divided into four stages or "plateaus." It's not merely the intensity that changes as the dose goes up, the effects change completely. At the lower plateaus, it's a stimulant with euphoric effects; at higher doses, it's a full on dissociative anesthetic, equally capable of producing sublime out-of-body experiences and episodes of temporary psychosis.

The Lower Plateaus

The lower plateaus are associated with euphoria and changes to the perception of sound and gravity. The first plateau produces fluid, "drippy" sensations, as though the body is a thick syrup. Most users react by adopting sweeping yet robotic movements as they navigate space. In this state, the user can still have conversations, and experienced psychonauts may enjoy this dosage at concerts or dance clubs, much like a low dose of ketamine.

Music may be especially pleasurable, an effect which is limited to the lower plateaus. "The music was more beautiful than I have ever heard," writes one user. Another describes an immersive musical landscape:

> The music totally pulled me in. I could no longer feel my body or the headphones. I felt like I was in some strange video game, flying over computer generated terrain. I often felt like I was in a huge concert hall listening to the music come from all around me. I was always in control, though. If I opened my eyes I could return to "reality."

According to William White, the author of an influential online guide to DXM, the pleasure produced by the substance

> . . . is totally unlike the euphoria from "body drugs" such as cocaine or heroin, and equally unlike the euphoria from MDMA (Ecstasy). Instead, it is a sensation of being totally at peace with oneself, the universe, and other people. Ordinary cares and concerns seem to vanish as one enters a world where anything is possible, and the body becomes increasingly irrelevant.

The second plateau intensifies the effects of the first, but adds some new features, such as closed-eye visual hallucinations and distortions to the fabric of time and space. The user becomes much more isolated from her environment, but is still coherent enough to interact with it. The senses start to flicker, as though all sounds and images are processed through a strobe light. Walking, dancing, and spinning become unusually pleasurable, thanks to physical sensations that mimic free-fall or low gravity.

Lower doses can also have empathogenic effects. Users often report a sense of empathy and openness that allows them to revisit old memories and confess secrets that would normally be too embarrassing to admit. Though likely less effective than MDMA in therapeutic contexts, this aspect of the DXM experience should not be overlooked. Therapeutic results may be limited by the compound's effects on memory: The higher the dose, the less one is likely to remember of the experience.

The Upper Plateaus

Higher doses should never be entered in a recreational context. These depths may contain significant value for someone with shamanic or exploratory intent, but casual users are bound to get more than they bargained for.

In the third plateau, the user becomes increasingly disconnected from the real world and can vividly experience scenes or memories conjured by the imagination. One is immersed in "weird, horizonless landscapes or spacescapes," and may feel as small as a molecule or as expansive as a galaxy. One explorer reports growing so large his head barely fit in the room and wore it as a helmet.

With eyes open, double vision prevails, as the brain refuses to resolve incoming visual data into a single three-dimensional image. The perceptual disturbances of the second plateau intensify: Both sights and sounds are divided into fragments that stutter through consciousness like Morse code telegrams. One experimenter says, "My visions were starting to freeze in place, as if everything were crystallizing or being coated in wax."

Although cognition is profoundly distorted, users also report a sense of serenity as distracting thoughts melt away. One person writes, "It felt like the top of my skull was opened into a clear blue sky."

The third plateau also marks the entrance of profound near-death and out-of-body experiences, which may be exhilarating, spiritually significant, or just plain terrifying. For these reasons, the third plateau is considered a serious and heavy trip. A hangover, consisting mostly of fatigue, is common.

In the fourth plateau, connection to "consensus reality" is totally cut off. A trip sitter—a sober companion who supervises the trip, keeps the subject from harming himself, and calls emergency services in case of overdose—is an absolute must. Proper dosing is critical: Overshooting the fourth plateau can result in a hospital stay or even death.

At this stage, the user is immersed in a full dissociative state, something like the "K-hole" of ketamine fame (see page 150). People frequently report encounters with God or other supernatural beings. Out-of-body experiences are common—perhaps even inevitable—but they can be deeply unnerving:

I imagined people sitting on my bed next to my body, and I had conversations with them from the other end of the room. I didn't actually talk out loud, because vocal sounds come from the body, and I had left it behind. . . . To me, I was dying. It was not scary, but just interesting. . . . It was incredibly powerful. A true spiritual pilgrimage.

In other descriptions of out-of-body experiences, the limits of language become painfully apparent. The person's interactions and sensations vary so profoundly from sober consciousness that they beggar the imagination.

I ended up in the middle of an endless mass of silver-golden light—I could feel every single particle of my being disintegrating and becoming part of the lightmass; indescribable sensations bombarded every part of me—far greater than any pleasure that I've experienced here on Earth.

But all is not warm and fuzzy. Higher plateaus frequently lead to delusional thinking, and brushes with psychosis are common. Although DXM is not particularly addictive, users who drink too deeply and too often from the trough of DXM consciousness run the risk of psychological addiction and other potential mental harms. Although relatively safe in the short term, the long-term consequences of DXM overuse are not well understood.

SPIRITUALITY AND "TRANSPERSONAL EXPERIENCES"

It may come as a surprise to the journalists, parents, and antidrug advocates who view the compound as little more than a social menace, but many people consider DXM an entheogen, or psychoactive sacrament. According to Dr. Peter Addy, a research scientist at Yale School of Medicine, DXM may be, "one of the few chemicals not currently under prohibition in the United States that facilitates access to transpersonal experiences."

For years, DXM users have remarked on its unusual ability to induce a variety of deeply meaningful experiences, ranging from the rekindling of long-forgotten childhood memories to exchanges with God, spirits, or other entities. Some descriptions are decidedly alien, made all the more fascinating by their detached matter-of-factness:

> *Gradually, these shifting forms were taking on more substance. They were coalescing into life forms; entities really—spectacular, bioluminescent, massy things that churned like thick, boiling, liquid. . . . Some were like complex blobs, jellyfish, or worms with thousands of pseudopodia. All were constantly writhing and huge. I could sense they were intelligent.*

> *. . . I never felt as if I were in danger. These things seemed not only friendly, but affectionate. . . . Their appearances were not monstrous so much as stunningly beautiful.*

Others take a more explicitly religious bent.

> *I felt as though I had a connection with God, one that I had never before had. . . . The upper plateaus are most definitely meant for spirituality I was being cradled by God as he protected me from myself. I was comforted, more than I ever had been before.*

Unpredictable and often challenging, the substance is one to be respected, perhaps even feared.

The sheer number of such powerful reactions makes one thing clear: DXM is much deeper and multifaceted than generally believed. Unpredictable and often challenging, the substance is one to be respected, perhaps even feared, but surely it deserves better than thoughtless demonization.

In spite of a half century of over-the-counter use, dextromethorphan's medical benefits have not yet been fully explored. Recent studies indicate it has neuroprotective properties that may prevent brain damage in a variety of critical situations, including fever, stroke, severe infection, and sudden injury.

Early research also shows promise at treating seizures, Parkinson's disease, shingles, and fibromyalgia among other conditions. It forms an ideal synergy with opioids such as morphine, potentiating their ability to kill pain while diminishing their addictive properties.

For a common cough medicine, DXM boasts a truly remarkable array of potential applications. Perhaps most ironic for a substance often seen as a "drug of abuse," DXM reduces withdrawal symptoms as well as tolerance to several addictive drugs, and, in the future, may play a significant role in treating drug addiction.

Given its therapeutic and spiritual potential, our culture's tendency to dismiss DXM consumption as "cough syrup abuse" appears embarrassingly narrow and unimaginative.

If circumstances were different—if, for instance, this synthetic chemical appeared in a mushroom or cactus and had been known to ancient peoples—it could easily stand among humanity's sacred medicines, revered for its visionary power and administered by skilled shamans in special ceremonies.

In the information age, debunking propaganda and myths takes only a few clicks of the mouse, and reliable information is more accessible than ever. Perhaps someday, this substance will shed its unglamorous reputation and take its place among the ranks of highly respected entheogens.

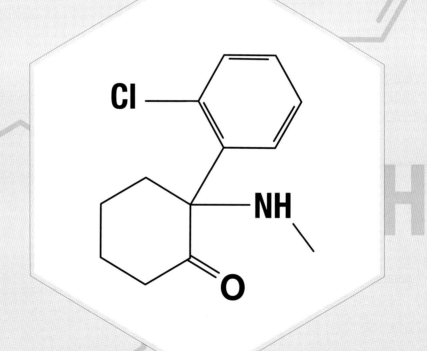

FIG. 3.2

(RS)-2-(2-CHLOROPHENYL)-2-(METHYLAMINO)CYCLOHEXANONE

DISCOVERED

Calvin Stevens at
Parke Davis Laboratories
in Detroit in 1962

KETAMINE

DURATION

up to 1 hour when insufflated
(sniffed) or injected; several
hours when ingested orally

ASSOCIATED WITH *rave and "clubbing" culture, veterinary and human medicine*

ORIGINS AND BACKGROUND

For a relative newcomer in the worlds of medicine and recreation, ketamine has made quite a splash. In just fifty years, ketamine has evolved from a promising anesthetic to a staple medicine in hospitals and veterinary clinics around the world, a sensation that overtook the clubbing and rave scenes, and an entheogen with serious self-exploratory potential. It also has a dark side: numbing, short-lived, and often euphoric, ketamine has drawn many into the spell of addiction. Chronic ketamine users frequently suffer kidney and bladder damage, among other health problems.

More recently, researchers have discovered in this anesthetic-cum-club-drug an unexpected hidden potential. Ketamine is now being studied as a medicine for some of our most stubborn mental illnesses, including depression and—ironically, for a compound that can lead to compulsive overuse—substance addiction. Like so many members of the psychedelic family, ketamine can be either a blessing or a curse, depending on the context and intention of use.

FROM PCP TO KETALAR

Calvin Stevens was a chemistry professor and pharmaceutical consultant when he stumbled upon ketamine in 1962. As a consultant to Parke Davis, at the time, America's oldest and largest pharmaceutical company now owned by Pfizer, Stevens synthesized a series of PCP derivatives in a search for the ideal anesthetic. In testing with monkeys, Parke Davis scientists determined that one of Stevens's PCP derivatives looked especially promising. Its chemical name is a mouthful: (RS)-2-(2-chlorophenyl)-2-(methylamino)cyclohexanone. Today, it's better known as ketamine.

Ketamine's appeal was manifold. Unlike most general anesthetics, it does not depress the patient's breathing, heart rate, or airway reflexes. When administered by medical personnel, it's remarkably safe, with a wide margin between a typical anesthetic dose and a toxic overdose. What makes ketamine truly unusual among anesthetics, though, is that it can be administered directly into muscle without having to find a vein. This quality recommends ketamine for use in emergency situations.

But ketamine was not a perfect medicine. The main problem was "emergence delirium"—as patients emerged from a deep anesthetic state, they complained of "strange experiences, like a feeling of floating in outer space and having no feeling in their arms or legs." Essentially, postoperative patients woke up tripping. It was hardly ideal, but compared to PCP and other lesser anesthetics, the symptoms were less severe and mercifully brief.

Though it had its shortcomings, the researchers had found their short-acting anesthetic. Ketamine became available under the brand name Ketalar in 1969.

FROM VIETNAM TO VETERINARY MEDICINE

Ketamine's first proving ground was the battlefield. It was used extensively as an emergency anesthetic by field medics in the Vietnam War. Some soldiers returned home with a taste for the stuff—perhaps it served to anesthetize not only war zone operations but mental traumas after the fact.

Recreational use began soon after Ketalar hit the market and grew slowly over the next two decades. Among recreational users, it would not really hit its stride until gaining massive popularity as a club drug in the 1990s.

Essentially, postoperative patients woke up tripping.

In the meantime, its appeal grew among veterinarians, who found in ketamine a safe and reliable anesthetic for a wide range of animals. It also became the top anesthetic in developing countries that lack resuscitation technology because it can be administered without slowing the heart or lungs. For regions with sophisticated health systems, however, its use has generally been limited to children and trauma patients, for whom alternative options may be too risky.

What prevented this purpose-built chemical from becoming the go-to medicine for all anesthetic needs? Its downfall was the emergence delirium that plagued postoperative patients with hallucinations and uncomfortable sensations. It turns out people getting surgeries prefer not to begin their recovery with a disturbing out-of-body experience.

But when it comes to using substances, humans are endlessly creative and motivated by many end goals. What the physician considers an undesirable side effect is regarded by psychonauts as the main event. Indeed, for some, the ketamine headspace represents the apex of all possible consciousness experiences. Anesthesia's loss is psychedelia's gain: Ketamine owes its enduring popularity among ravers and consciousness explorers to the same qualities doctors struggle to suppress.

Nevertheless, because of its safety profile and ease of administration, it is still considered a staple drug in medicine. The World Health Organization lists it as one of its "essential medicines," the fundamental drugs that hospitals across the world must stock to meet the basic needs of their patients. And in veterinary clinics, ketamine remains the primary anesthetic for all species. Apparently, no one is worried about Lassie suffering from a postoperative dissociative episode.

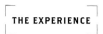

THE EXPERIENCE

The synthesis of ketamine is quite complex, so the black market supply is most often diverted from legitimate sources—often pharmaceutical companies in India or Mexico—rather than produced in clandestine labs. It is typically snorted as a white powder. In liquid form, it can also be injected into a muscle or, less commonly, directly into a vein. By injection, the ketamine experience is shorter, more intense, and comes on more quickly.

Edward Domino, who conducted the first human trials of ketamine, was unsure how to characterize the substance. When the professor described the "disconnection" felt by his research subjects to his wife, Toni, she suggested the term "dissociative anesthetic." The name has stuck.

For millions of people, ketamine represents the definitive dissociative experience. At low doses, it can be stimulating and even sociable, as many thousands of clubbers and ravers can attest. Physical sensations also change—the sense of proportions of one's body can shrink or elongate, coordination is compromised, and movements take on a "bouncy" quality that encourages sweeping, exaggerated gestures. A survey of ketamine users found that their favorite aspects were hallucinations, giddiness, out-of-body experiences, and "melting into the surroundings." With a push of energy, distortions of time and space, and an indescribable "dreamy" feeling, many find it ideal for a night out dancing.

Care must be taken not to overindulge, however, or a partygoer is liable to wind up on the floor, uncommunicative, while his astral form roams the cosmos. At higher doses, the trip becomes deeply introspective. This dosage precludes any coherent connection with reality and is completely incompatible with the dance scene. Those who choose to venture this far opt for more private environments.

THE K-HOLE AND THE NEAR-DEATH EXPERIENCE

In a full dissociative state, or "K-hole," the user appears almost comatose to an outside observer. Yet inside, the person may be in the throes of ecstasy or of despair, exploring hidden recesses of the mind or even reliving birth. Having shed the body like an old snakeskin, there is no telling where the mind may wander. Dissociation has two major components: *depersonalization*—the feeling of detaching from one's self or body and viewing it from an outside perspective; and *derealization*, the conviction that reality is not quite real, but rather a simulation, projection, or lucid dream.

These dissociative qualities distort consciousness in fundamental ways. Our everyday experience is rooted in a sense of selfhood—the constant, abiding presence we call "I"—and in the steady, reliable "realness" of our surrounding environment. With those anchors lifted, consciousness becomes fluid and abstract, floating like an astronaut untethered in space. Everything—objects, friends, even the user's own emotions and thoughts—becomes distant, as though observed by a neutral third party. Time stands still, and all awareness appears to condense into a universal singularity.

JOHN C. LILLY

Neuroscientist, author, and psychedelic enthusiast John C. Lilly was a man of many interests and wild ideas. A lifelong explorer of consciousness, Lilly never hesitated to dive headfirst into any subject that piqued his boundless curiosity, even when that meant using his own mind as an experimental laboratory.

Dedicated to his work and more than a little eccentric, Lilly fit neatly into the popular archetype of "mad scientist." He is perhaps best remembered for his research with dolphins, who he believed could communicate with humans—if only we could decipher their unique language of squeaks and clicks.

But Lilly was also an avid explorer of inner space, exemplifying the term "psychonaut" long before it gained popular currency. He invented the isolation tank—a totally enclosed sensory-deprivation chamber filled with buoyant, body-temperature water. Designed to remove all sensation of sight, sound, and touch, the isolation tank separates the mind from the physical self, producing a substance-free form of dissociation.

Lilly also experimented with high doses of LSD and ketamine, documenting the results in several autobiographical books. He often combined these chemical experiments with his other research interests, spending many hours telepathically communicating with

dolphins or exploring the seemingly limitless bounds of his mind while floating in one of his tanks.

Lilly became an alarmingly frequent user of ketamine, occasionally injecting it every hour for days at a time. He claimed the substance provided a window into other realities:

On K . . . I can open my eyes in this reality and dimly see the alternate reality, then close my eyes, and the alternate reality picks up. On K you can tune your internal eyes.

On two different occasions, he nearly died from reckless overuse of the substance, and he began to elaborate bizarre conspiracy theories about cosmic entities who interfere in human affairs. In spite of his excesses—or perhaps because of them—his books gained a significant readership and exposed ketamine to a broader audience. Today, John Lilly's writings provide a fascinating insight into the incredible power, and very real dangers, of a human mind immersed in ketamine space.

The dissociative state shares many qualities with classic near-death experiences: floating outside the body and observing it from above, transcending reality and receiving secret insights about the meaning of existence, and having one's life "flash before your eyes," a vivid review of forgotten memories some people find therapeutic. In spite of the name, a person need not be in any physical danger to have such a near-death experience.

One of the most fascinating connections is the appearance of spiritual connotations in both ketamine and near-death experiences, even in nonreligious people. Travelers to deep inner space sometimes speak of surrendering to God, entering a bright internal light, or falling through a formless void, where they become filled with an ineffable sense of serenity and oneness.

THE RISE AND EVOLUTION OF KETAMINE CULTURE

Though there had always been enthusiastic psychonauts in the style of John Lilly, ketamine did not really become popular outside the field of medicine until the 1990s when it exploded onto the clubbing and rave scenes. There, amid the throngs of bodies, vibrant lights, and thumping bass, this tranquilizer found a new home.

Ketamine first emerged as an adulterant in pills sold as Ecstasy, but soon become popular in its own right. At that time, ketamine had not been scheduled as an illegal drug and remained legally available from chemical supply companies and online sources. Before long, ketamine had made the jump from the rave subculture to mainstream popularity.

Naturally, hysteria ensued. The media painted it as the new drug menace, printing sensationalized reports of overdoses and exaggerating its use as a date rape drug. In fact, overdoses from pure ketamine are very rare, as are cases of sexual assault resulting from its unwitting use. Alcohol remains the most widely used date rape drug, by a tremendous margin. Nevertheless, the devil had to be exorcised, and, in 1999, the government classified ketamine as a controlled substance.

Prohibition has done little to dent its momentum, however. An estimated 2.7 million Americans have tried ketamine in their lifetime, and today it remains a popular choice among both casual clubbers and dedicated psychonauts around the world.

THE DARK SIDE OF KETAMINE

What begins as an experiment in consciousness or a weekend binge can escalate into addiction. Although the majority of ketamine users never become dependent, for some, it grows into a compulsive diversion. Within weeks, some people find themselves consuming several grams every day. Though fatal overdoses are extremely rare, ketamine has been implicated in many deaths through reckless behavior including car crashes, drownings, and overdoses from unsafe combinations with other drugs such as alcohol or benzodiazepines.

When used alone without proper precautions, ketamine can result in accidental death by incapacitating the user in a dangerous situation. It should never be used in high doses without a trusted sober "sitter" who can supervise the session and react appropriately to an emergency.

Chronic ketamine use also causes physical damage, in particular, problems with the urinary tract including cysts, incontinence, painful urination, and blood in the urine. Regular use also takes a mental toll and can interfere with memory, sleep, and emotional health. Ketamine is a dissociative anesthetic in more ways than one—chronic use can isolate a person from friends and loved ones, and can numb emotional pain. When it is used in this way, ketamine is not an entheogen but a dangerous and solitary distraction.

Ketamine did not really become popular outside the field of medicine until the 1990s when it exploded onto the clubbing and rave scenes.

Even with a well-established medical staple like ketamine, our scientific understanding keeps evolving. New research continues to untangle this molecular mystery, revealing several potential new treatment angles. Ketamine has demonstrated surprising effectiveness in treating a number of tough-to-crack conditions including alcoholism, opioid addiction, chronic pain, and, in particular, chronic depression.

Ketamine psychotherapy as a treatment for alcoholism appears very promising. Altogether more than a thousand alcoholic patients have been treated with ketamine without any lasting adverse reactions. In one study conducted by the Russian psychiatrist Evgeny Krupitsky with more than two hundred alcohol-dependent subjects, 65 percent of those treated with ketamine remained abstinent a full year later, compared with 24 percent of the control group. Thorough preparation and post-trip integration, in which the patients reflect on the meaning of their ketamine session, are critical to the success of this type of therapy.

Though effective, it was not easy. Patients reported, "diverse experiences ranging from spiritual rapture to fear and even horror." For the subjects, the positive effects demonstrated the potential of a sober lifestyle, and the fearful parts, a visceral demonstration of their own toxic relationship with alcohol.

A similar approach has also been taken with addiction to opioids and cocaine. Heroin-dependent individuals treated with "ketamine psychedelic therapy," or KPT, showed a higher incidence of abstinence than those treated with traditional psychotherapy after two years. Another study conducted by Dr. Krupitsky showed that with three sessions of KPT, heroin-dependent people were more than twice as likely to remain abstinent one year later than those who had a single session.

In more recent studies, ketamine has shown promise as a potential treatment for obsessive-compulsive disorder and post-traumatic stress disorder. A small

Altogether more than a thousand alcoholic patients have been treated with ketamine without any lasting adverse reactions.

proof-of-concept study showed that ketamine may offer relief for those with social anxiety disorder, with a single dose reducing anxiety for up to two weeks. It can also help those with chronic pain manage with lower doses of opioids— a blessing, considering the addictive and sedating qualities of opioid painkillers. More commonly, ketamine has become a choice medicine for various types of severe neuropathic pain, including phantom limb pain, an excruciating and obstinate condition suffered by most amputees.

Of ketamine's many promising new uses, the most notable is for depression. A host of studies reveal that a single low dose of ketamine reduces depression within hours, even in those who have not responded well to talk therapy, antidepressants, or other medications. Relief lasts up to a week. Suicidal tendencies are also greatly reduced. Researchers are unsure how ketamine induces such long-lived benefits, as the active compound is eliminated from the body in a matter of hours.

These early and somewhat surprising results suggest ketamine may offer benefits for a wider variety of clinical applications than anyone had previously guessed. If this humble tranquilizer continues to astound, it will be a very long time before our understanding of it is complete.

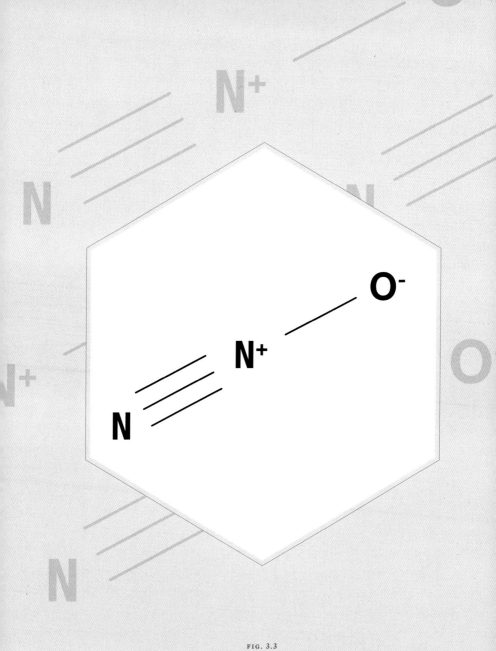

FIG. 3.3

N_2O

NITROUS OXIDE

ALSO KNOWN AS *laughing gas*

ORIGINS AND BACKGROUND

THE SMALLEST AND SIMPLEST OF ALL PSYCHEDELIC CHEMICALS, nitrous oxide is simply an oxygen atom attached to two nitrogens. It's a transparent, odorless gas with a faintly sweet taste. Known as laughing gas, it's been widely used in dentistry since 1844 and boasts an even longer history of recreational use. And yet today, nearly two and a half centuries after its discovery, exactly how it elicits its painkilling, euphoric, and dissociative effects remains something of a mystery.

Nitrous oxide, or N_2O, was discovered in 1772 by the natural philosopher Sir Joseph Priestley, who called it, "dephlogisticated nitrous air." It caused a sensation when it was introduced to upper-crust society in late-eighteenth-century London. Aristocrats gathered for "laughing gas parties" and got high through elaborate contraptions that looked more like chemistry sets than drug paraphernalia. For decades it was known only as a novelty, a gaseous gateway to strange realms of consciousness that attracted scientists, philosophers, and plain old partying Englishmen.

Today, the gas bears an abundance of uses and is as likely to be encountered in a dentist's office as a professional kitchen or a race car's gas tank. Outside of medicine, its main uses are culinary—for dessert caterers, it is the go-to substance for making a voluminous whipped cream—and automotive—popular as a fuel additive for race cars, nitrous oxide has also been implemented in the engines of rockets and airplanes. It's even a natural component of our atmosphere, but at 0.33 parts per million, the only high you're likely to get from huffing fresh air is from hyperventilation.

One good lungful provides a 30-second experience characterized by instant euphoria, dissociative sensations of detachment, and distinctive, echoing audio distortions often described as "flanging." Tingles run through the body, and users often become lightheaded and lose their balance. Higher doses can lead to out-of-body experiences and fully immersive hallucinations, but rarely last longer than a couple minutes.

It's especially common at music festivals, where seated circles of youths pass around brightly colored balloons filled with the gaseous elixir. About one in twenty Americans has tried N_2O at some point.

One compelling report of the experience comes from a most unlikely source. Eight years before he became prime minister of the United Kingdom, Winston Churchill was searching for a friend's house in New York City. Accustomed to the left-hand drivers of London, he looked the wrong way when crossing Fifth Avenue and was hit by a passing car. In the hospital, he was administered nitrous oxide.

Churchill did not enjoy the process. By his description, the trauma of the car crash almost seems preferable:

> *With me the nitrous-oxide trance usually takes this form: The sanctum is occupied by alien powers. I see the absolute truth and explanation of things, but something is left out which upsets the whole . . . This almost breaks mortal comprehension. It is beyond anything the human mind was ever meant to master.*

> *The process continues inexorably. Depth beyond depth of unendurable truth opens. I have, therefore, always regarded the nitrous-oxide trance as a mere substitution of mental for physical pain.*

For others, this "depth beyond depth" of truth is one of nitrous oxide's best features.

But those who've delved the deepest—from Sir Humphry Davy to William James—remark on the ineffable, metaphysical breadth of the nitrous experience.

NO LAUGHING MATTER: RISK AND DANGERS

Nitrous oxide is among the safest and least addictive of all recreational substances. Nevertheless, some people do become hooked, and others have died from reckless use of the gas.

Deaths from nitrous oxide almost always involve unsafe practices such as gasmasks, bags, or enclosed spaces, which greatly increase the risk of suffocation. In medical contexts, nitrous is administered along with equal parts oxygen to ensure healthy respiration. Recreational users inhale pure nitrous oxide, temporarily depriving the body of oxygen. As long as the user breathes fresh air regularly—and cannot, in the event of passing out, become trapped in an enclosed environment—this does not pose a major threat.

Because the gas cools rapidly as it expands, inhaling it directly from a canister can cause serious throat burns. And because it compromises the sense of balance, falls are fairly common. It doesn't take a consultation with an anesthesiologist to realize this is a substance best served seated.

In spite of these risks, nitrous oxide remains a remarkably nontoxic substance when ingested responsibly. Inhaling laughing gas from a balloon eliminates most practical risks. Maybe it's a good sign the colorful latex globes have become the calling card of the nitrous oxide subculture, brightening the fields of festivals where metaphysically minded people gather.

THE DISCOVERY OF NITROUS OXIDE

One thinks of recreational nitrous use as a modern phenomenon and as a diversion from its "legitimate" uses in dentist's offices and whipped cream canisters. Yet, the first "trip reports" on laughing gas may well represent the birth of psychedelic literature in the West, appearing a good century and a half before Leary, Huxley, and Kesey ever picked up a pen. And its appeal as a dental anesthetic emerged from its utility as a mental exploration tool, not the other way around.

About one in twenty Americans has tried N_2O at some point.

When he discovered nitrous oxide in 1772, the English chemist Sir Joseph Priestley was no stranger to science. Though most famous for the discovery of oxygen, he made a variety of contributions to philosophy, chemistry, and electricity. To top it off, he even invented a novel method of carbonating water. But although he enjoyed the refreshing taste of soda water, he was never tempted to sample his other gaseous creations. The discovery of nitrous oxide's psychoactive properties would have to wait for more adventurous—or reckless—explorers.

In 1799, a physician named Thomas Beddoes established a medical research facility in Bristol, England, dedicated to treating patients with medicinal gases. He called it the Pneumatic Institution, and as its superintendent he hired Humphry Davy, a brilliant young chemist and inventor.

Nitrous oxide became a prime focus for Davy and the Pneumatic Institution. Unlike Priestley, Davy had no qualms about inhaling novel gases—that was, after all, the whole point of the Institution. Davy imbibed nitrous oxide with a passion that others reserved for more common inebriants such as alcohol, tobacco, and opium and eventually became addicted to it. "I have often felt very great pleasure," he wrote, "when breathing it alone, in darkness and silence, occupied only by ideal existence."

THE PNEUMATIC INSTITUTION

In its early days, nitrous oxide attracted not dentists and surgeons, but creative and curious spirits—poets and philosophers, as well as scientists and inventors. Enamored with the novel state of mind he had uncovered, Davy introduced laughing gas to many of his contemporaries, including James Watt, Peter Mark Roget, and the Romantic poets Robert Southey and Samuel Taylor Coleridge. Davy began hosting what might be called the first-ever psychedelic parties, and his circle of friends offered their impressions of this unique inebriant.

After extensive experimentation with the gas, Davy penned a six hundred-page tract collecting the results of his intense and frequent experiences. Published in 1800, the book included subjective reports from many of those who passed through the Institution's doors. Samuel Coleridge described the high as a "pleasurable sensation of warmth over my whole frame, resembling what I remember once to have experienced after returning from a walk in the snow into a warm room." Peter Mark Roget was less descriptive. "I felt myself totally incapable of speaking," he said—a striking sentiment, coming from the man who would later pen the quintessential writer's tool, *Roget's Thesaurus*.

James Watt is best known as the namesake of the unit of electrical energy, the *watt*, and inventor of the steam engine that made the Industrial Revolution possible. But he also made a unique contribution to the Pneumatic Institute, designing a portable version of Davy's inhalation chamber to facilitate easier consumption.

In the course of their experiments, Davy and Dr. Beddoes made a prescient observation. Noting that cuts stopped hurting while intoxicated with nitrous oxide, they surmised the gas had painkilling properties. Davy correctly predicted its use as a surgical anesthetic, but, as usual, he was ahead of his time—the medical world took another forty years to catch on.

THE PHILOSOPHER PSYCHONAUT
WILLIAM JAMES

Another luminary to plumb the depths of nitrous consciousness was William James, the father of American psychology and author of several influential texts on philosophy and the human mind. James was especially interested in altered states of consciousness and wrote at length about the importance of mystical experiences. One of his greatest achievements was wrangling spirituality into the realm of psychology, legitimizing "religious experiences" under the banner of science—all by way of altered states of mind, which he considered essential to the study of human spirituality.

After experimenting with copious amounts of laughing gas, James was floored. "With me, as with every other person of whom I have heard," he wrote, "the keynote of the experience is the tremendously exciting sense of an intense metaphysical illumination."

The revelations were not easy to articulate. Overcome by his mystical experiences, he scrawled endless sheets of bizarre phrases and thoughts.

"What's mistake but a kind of take?" wrote the nitrous-addled philosopher. Indeed, "What's nausea but a kind of -ausea? . . . Agreement—disagreement!! Emotion—motion!!"

Sound crazy? James agreed, but chalked it up to the ineffable nature of the experience: "That sounds like nonsense, but it's pure *on* sense! Thought much deeper than speech. . . !"

In nitrous oxide's early days, it was viewed more as a novelty than a medical breakthrough. By the early 1800s, the well-to-do were gathering for "laughing gas parties," and N_2O became a popular demonstration tool for traveling hucksters.

In 1844, a dentist named Horace Wells attended a "Grand Exhibition" of the gas's exhilarating effects in Connecticut. During the demonstration, Wells watched as an inebriated attendee fell, injuring himself but showing no sign of pain.

Wells immediately realized the gas's potential as a surgical anesthetic. The very next day, he arranged to have one of his teeth pulled under the influence of nitrous oxide—the first ever use of laughing gas in a dental surgery.

Before long, Wells was using nitrous oxide on patients in his private dental practice. Eager to share the newfound anesthetic with the wider medical community, he arranged a series of demonstrations where he would perform the impossible for a skeptical audience, extracting patients' teeth without any pain at all.

But success eluded him. When an error resulted in a patient crying out in pain at a demonstration to Boston medical students in 1845, the crowd booed. Devastated, Wells returned to Hartford, where he soon shuttered his dental practice. Three years later, living alone and addicted to chloroform and ether, he took his own life.

Wells's dream did come true in the end, and today, Wells is honored as the pioneer of surgical anesthesia. Though recognition came too late to make a difference in his lifetime, Wells's discovery has lessened the suffering of countless people all over the world.

IS LAUGHING GAS THE BEST MEDICINE?

Of the three original gaseous anesthetics, only nitrous oxide remains in use today. The others, ether and chloroform, have long since given way to safer and more effective agents. The use of nitrous oxide also decreased with the advent of longer-lasting anesthetics in the 1950s, but never disappeared entirely. Though once the leading anesthetic for labor pains, nitrous oxide gradually fell by the wayside in the United States as the epidural needle became all the rage.

N_2O is still widely used in dentistry, where its chief purpose is to sedate and relieve anxiety before the administration of a more powerful anesthetic. Emergency services also use nitrous oxide to quell pain and anxiety while en route to a hospital. And it has remained useful as a sedative in pediatric medicine, thanks to its low toxicity and ease of administration.

In Europe and Canada, where its use in childbirth never waned, it remains a popular choice for labor pain relief. It's cheap, extremely fast acting, and safe for both mother and child. Best of all, it can be self-administered—the mother can place the mask over her face as contractions begin and remove it as necessary. No other pain management solution offers such complete and immediate control to the patient. In some progressive American hospitals, laughing gas is officially back on the menu for women in labor.

N_2O has also emerged as an unlikely medicine for several mental health issues, including substance withdrawal and depression. A 2015 study showed that, in a small sample of people with treatment-resistant depression for whom none of the traditional approaches, including antidepressants and talk therapy, had much effect, one in five experienced significant relief after inhaling nitrous oxide.

It has also been examined as an acute treatment for alcohol withdrawal. Compared to the best current treatment options—Valium and similar drugs—nitrous oxide appears to act more quickly and be just as effective.

From a chemical curiosity in the 1770s to a philosophical tool in 1800, the gas remained little more than a novelty among the elite for the next half century. As its anesthetic effects were realized, it became a medical sensation overnight, though it eventually fell from favor as more powerful anesthetics became available. And now, a full two and a half centuries after "dephlogisticated nitrous air" was first discovered, it is once again turning heads in medicine.

Since the early days of Humphry Davy, there have been philosophers, poets, and seekers of all types, breathing the gas for decidedly nonmedical purposes—whether transcendence, inspiration, or simple curiosity. The trend will surely continue as long as human intellect is stirred to reach beyond earthbound life, to be buoyed to upper atmospheres of consciousness on currents of laughing gas.

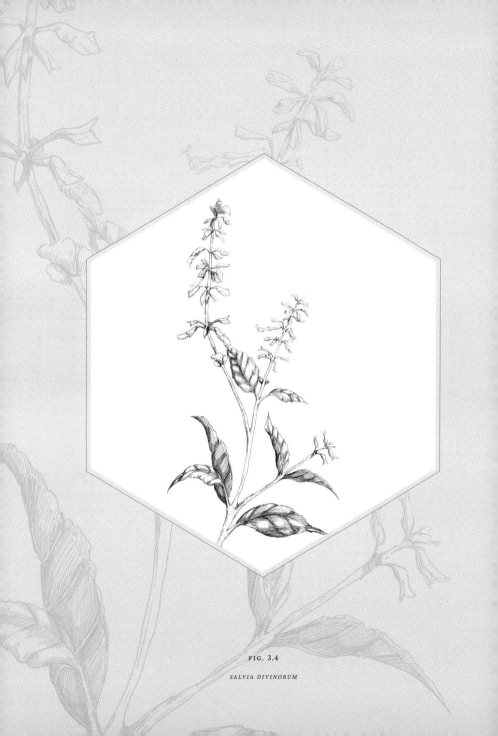

FIG. 3.4

SALVIA DIVINORUM

DISCOVERED

Use by the Mazatec dates
back centuries, possibly
even millennia

DURATION

15 minutes to 2 hours

SALVIA

ASSOCIATED WITH *Mazatec people of Oaxaca, Mexico*

KEY COMPOUNDS *Salvinorin A*

ORIGINS AND BACKGROUND

AMONG PSYCHOACTIVE PLANTS, *SALVIA DIVINORUM* is utterly unique. Though it's a member of the mint family and a close relative of common sage, salvia—or "diviner's sage," as its Latin name translates—packs far more of a punch than these kitchen staples. In fact, its active ingredient, Salvinorin A, is the most potent psychoactive compound in all of nature. It's often classed as a dissociative alongside ketamine and DXM, but its effects stand in a league of their own.

A striking example of the power of cultural beliefs, salvia means two very different things to the two cultures where it is encountered. To the Mazatec, an indigenous people based in the mountains of southern Mexico, salvia is a treasured plant spirit who imparts healing knowledge to learned shamans. It has a long history of use and is approached with utmost respect to ascertain answers to important questions. Because it is usually made into a water infusion, and never smoked, it induces a serene trance state that lasts for 1 or 2 hours.

To modern Western users, who first encountered this peculiar plant in recent decades, salvia represents little more than a novelty. Though there is a handful of salvia devotees who use it as a spiritual tool, the plant is usually sought for its unique high in the name of simple curiosity. It's even been marketed as a marijuana substitute, but, in reality, the two plants have little in common other than being psychoactive and green.

In recent years, salvia has emerged as the unlikely star of a number of online videos featuring teenagers smoking a highly concentrated form of the herb and then stumbling over furniture while slurring words or laughing uncontrollably. It's fair to say the typical American approach to salvia is both more intense and less informed than that of their counterparts south of the border. As a result, it has earned a negative reputation in the media and in the minds of concerned parents —a fact that would shock the Mazatec shamans who have passed knowledge of this sacred plant down for countless generations.

THE MAZATEC MEDICINE

Because of the influence of Christian colonialism, it's impossible to determine what the Mazatec salvia ritual may have looked like in pre-Columbian times. The Mazatec's many names for salvia, including *hoja de la Pastora* or *ska Pastora*— the shepherdess's leaf—and *yerba de Maria*—the herb of Mary—demonstrate the remarkable influence of Catholicism on this native tradition.

The seer's sage is always taken at night, in a place of silence and stillness. The shaman sits alone with the patient, administers the proper dose, and intones prayers that combine both traditional and Christian themes, calling upon the Holy Trinity and the Virgin Mary as well as the gods of the rainforest and the sun.

Both the healer and the patient ingest the leaves or tea and enter a trance state. The session may be sought for more than just medical reasons—if an item is lost, salvia will help find it; if the subject has been the victim of a theft or witchcraft, salvia will identify the culprit; and if the person simply needs guidance and direction, salvia will provide it.

María Sabina, the Mazatec healer who unwittingly unleashed psilocybin mushrooms upon the world by sharing them with R. Gordon Wasson, considered salvia a secondary entheogen. "When I am in the time that there are no mushrooms and want to heal someone who is sick," she explained, "then I must fall back on the leaves of *Pastora*." Ground up and swallowed, she added, they worked just like the mushrooms—yet nowhere near as powerful.

Given that salvia leaves contain the most potent hallucinogen in nature, that assessment comes as a surprise. The perceived lack of potency is best explained by the Mazatec's preferred methods of consumption—either drinking a thick green tea or chewing fresh leaves, absorbing the active compounds through the gums and cheeks before swallowing. Though time-honored traditions, these are actually the least efficient ways of consuming salvia and produce a much subtler and longer-lasting effect than the typical Western method of smoking the leaves.

SCIENCE AND SALVIA

Few visionary plants have managed to maintain a veil of secrecy for as long as salvia. The Mazatec have probably been using salvia for centuries, but the plant and its stunning effects remained unknown to science until the twentieth century. In 1939, anthropologist Jean Bassett Johnson studied Mazatec shamanism and became the first to reveal this mysterious plant to the world. He collected a few

THE MOST POTENT PSYCHEDELIC IN NATURE

Salvia's active compound, Salvinorin A, remained unknown until 1982. The most potent psychoactive substance in nature, as little as a half milligram of Salvinorin A can send you on a psychedelic voyage. But even aside from its incredible potency, Salvinorin A is an unusual specimen. For twenty years, scientists were stumped as to how exactly the chemical exerts its effects upon the brain. Typical psychedelics, such as psilocybin and LSD, act on the brain's serotonin receptors. Dissociatives, such as ketamine, PCP, and DXM (cough medicine), act primarily by blocking a key excitatory chemical in the brain called NMDA. But Salvinorin A has no affinity for serotonin or NMDA receptors.

Researchers finally figured it out in 2002. Salvinorin A works its magic by triggering a particular type of opioid receptor called the KOR, the kappa opioid receptor. It is the only substance found in nature to act selectively on this receptor, which helps explain its singularly bizarre qualities. Its profound effects have led some scientists to speculate that KOR—and the claustrum, a region of the brain where these receptors are most densely expressed—are fundamental to our experience of everyday consciousness.

of its leaves and even tried the brew himself, proving the jungle plant was more than mere myth. Unfortunately, Johnson's research was interrupted by World War II.

The seer's sage would have to wait several more decades for its day in the sun. In 1962, mycologist R. Gordon Wasson and chemist Albert Hofmann returned from Oaxaca with the first ever-flowering samples of the shrub. Their colleague and botanist Carl Epling identified it as a new species, dubbing it *Salvia divinorum*—the diviner's sage.

THE EXPERIENCE

The salvia experience features some of the typical dissociative effects, such as profound distortions of one's sense of self and what constitutes reality, but ultimately it stands in a class of its own. Though it offers powerful visual and bodily hallucinations, they are not remotely similar to those of classical psychedelics such as LSD or psilocybin mushrooms. Far from euphoric, the salvia headspace tends to be bleaker and more disturbing than the more popular psychedelics. But for a select group of devotees who celebrate the plant's placid and even spiritual effects, there is no better "plant teacher" than *Salvia divinorum*.

Physical sensations such as pulling, stretching, or flying are common. Users frequently feel as though they are sinking into the furniture, or even falling through the floor altogether, watching it drift away as they descend into ever-stranger realms. Salvia fiddles with fundamental levers in our brain's sense of identity: People often report merging into nearby inanimate objects, discarding their human forms like snakeskins as they embrace their new—albeit short-lived—lives as chairs, walls, or carpets.

Common themes include tunnels and spirals, with people often feeling like reality itself is peeling apart. Occasionally, salvia offers contact with "entities" or spirits who may guide the user through the experience.

Seconds after smoking the potent leaves, it's easy to forget one has taken a substance at all, and all preconceptions—relationships, histories, names, all the things that make us human—sink away, replaced by the inexplicable realization that *this is reality now*. For a few short minutes, the user remains lost in these rarefied corridors of consciousness. Then, thankfully, sobriety returns, and, along with it, one's sense of self—miraculously intact.

On Erowid, the online drug library, a user going by Temicxoch does an admirable job of wrangling the ineffable experience into words:

> I closed my eyes and lost all sense of my physical self. I roared through a void. I was surrounded by a space of myriad expanse, yet there was nothing there. I was exploding in all directions at once, expanding, twisting outward, yet there was nothing through which to be moving. I flew, I floated, I flourished. The dark matter which filled me and which I encompassed sang with energy. Just as the abyss about me had a form, so its silence was an ecstatic polyphony. My senses rang with delight.

For some, the experience can feel "more real than reality," and people sometimes emerge from the salvia spell with the impression that a veil has been temporarily lifted. The unsettling conclusion—that one's whole life has been nothing but a dream, or a simulation—sometimes leads to an existential freak-out or identity crisis. Thankfully, these feelings usually wear off on their own.

ADDICTIVE DRUG OR VISIONARY BALM?

It comes as no surprise that, in such a state, a salvia user's coordination becomes compromised. A regular living room becomes fraught with obstacles as the inebriated person is tugged by unseen forces, hopelessly adrift in an unfamiliar intersection of time and space. To avoid injury, it's critical to have a trip sitter.

And yet, in spite of what videos of stumbling, tongue-tied youths may suggest, the experience is really nothing like being drunk. The salvia spell keeps its target in a heightened state of awareness, fully cognizant of a compelling alternate reality even as balance and language disappear into the void.

Far from euphoric, the salvia headspace tends to be bleaker and more disturbing than the more popular psychedelics.

Like other powerful psychoactive substances, salvia can leave some users with lasting feelings of anxiety and must be approached carefully. Yet, because of its decidedly noneuphoric effects, it has a very low risk of dependence. In fact, its effects on the brain are the exact opposite of those that light up our "reward network," such as cocaine and methamphetamine.

For the vast majority of people, salvia usage tapers off naturally—after a strong first dose, many swear it off for good. The herb's self-regulating nature has probably helped it remain legal in cultures where most intoxicants, aside from alcohol and tobacco, are vehemently suppressed.

And yet, even this is changing—in the wake of media attention highlighting examples of careless use, tolerance for the plant has waned. Though federally unregulated, salvia is now illegal in a majority of states, making it the latest victim of the war on inebriants and visionary medicines begun by the first colonists of this continent.

Meanwhile, in Oaxaca, the diviner's sage lives on as a vital component of daily life—a balm for many ailments, a source of answers in times of uncertainty, and a dose of serenity in a world of chaos. It's hard to believe that American commentators and Mazatec shamans are speaking of the same plant.

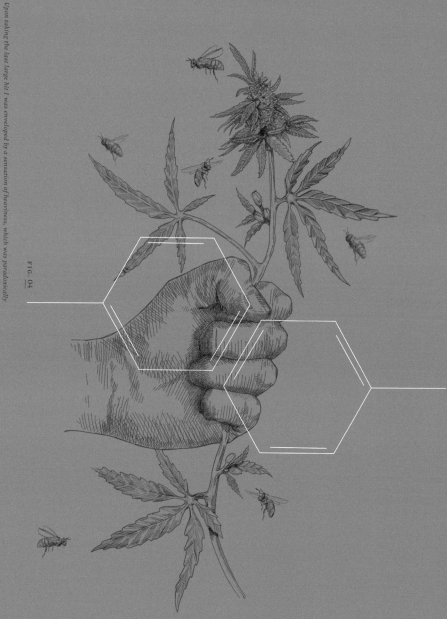

FIG. 04

Upon taking the last large hit I was enveloped by a sensation of heaviness, which was paradoxically light and spacious. . . . My head and hands felt as though they could detach and float away from my body . . . At another point I felt as though gravity had changed in a similar manner that one would experience while submerged in water

CHAPTER FOUR

UNIQUE PSYCHEDELICS

The psychedelic misfits, united not by what they have in common, but by how they stand apart. From the speckled *Amanita* mushroom in snowy Siberia to the green "ganja" of Indian mystics; from intoxicating honey gathered from towering Himalayan cliffs to sponges growing at the bottom of the sea—these substances are among the strangest known to man.

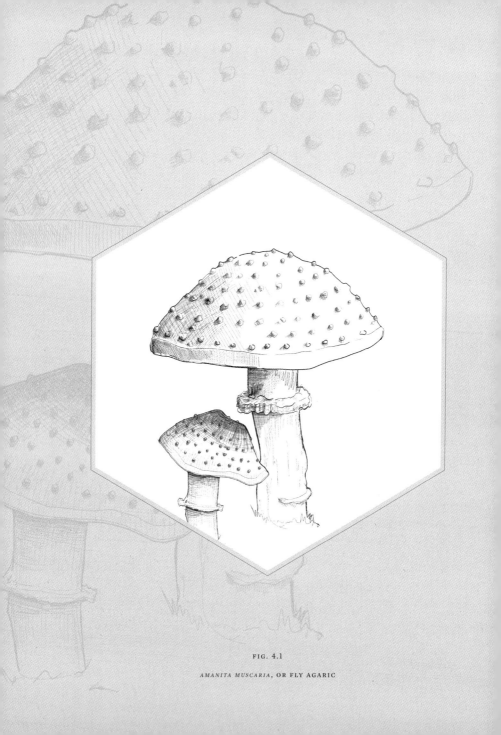

FIG. 4.1

AMANITA MUSCARIA, OR FLY AGARIC

DISCOVERED

Known to Siberian shamans
for millennia; first discovered
by Europeans in the early
1700s

AMANITA MUSCARIA

DURATION

6 to 8 hours

ASSOCIATED WITH *traditional Siberian cultures*

KEY COMPOUNDS *muscimol, ibotenic acid*

ORIGINS AND BACKGROUND

*A*MANITA MUSCARIA, OR FLY AGARIC, BOASTS what may be the most conspicuous and iconic appearance of all psychoactive life forms. Gathered in quaint bunches under evergreens or birches, *Amanita*'s bright red caps sprinkled with white polka dots form an unmistakable, almost surreal, image. One almost expects to see garden fairies flitting about this idyllic scene, but, of course, they're not likely to appear until after the mushroom is consumed.

Over the centuries, *Amanita muscaria* has emerged as pop culture's archetypal mushroom, making an appearance in everything from gnome-laden garden ornaments and kitschy knickknacks to videogame power-ups and children's books. Two of Disney's classic films, *Fantasia* and *Snow White*, feature the iconic mushroom in scenes of lively dancing, reminiscent of its traditional use among Far Eastern shamans.

The mushroom's enduring popularity in modern times probably owes more to its striking appearance and global distribution than its mental effects. It's doubtful whether something as innocuous as the Smurfs' toadstool houses represents a deliberate allusion to drug-induced visions. Nevertheless, its association with magic, fairies, and spirits persists to this day.

Long before it invaded popular consciousness, *A. muscaria* first spread its fibrous tendrils across the physical world. For millennia, it was utilized for both religious and recreational purposes by traditional cultures in Siberia. From there, it expanded through Asia, Europe, and North America. Today, it can be found all over the world, though in some areas it is considered an invasive species—more fungal weed than gift of the gods.

Wherever it grows, it forms a symbiotic relationship with a host tree—a mutually beneficial arrangement where the fungus colonizes and extends the tree's root system. Because of this, the mushroom cannot be cultivated, only harvested in the wild. The host trees are typically birches or pines, but *A. muscaria* isn't choosy. In Australia, it even allies itself with eucalyptus trees—a far cry from the snowy pines of its homeland. It's something of a fungal stowaway, with spores that readily voyage across oceans by clinging to the seeds of imported trees.

The *Amanita* genus includes perfectly edible species, along with some of the most poisonous mushrooms on the planet, including the Destroying Angels and Death Caps, which are responsible for more than 90 percent of all mushroom-induced fatalities. The two most famous psychoactive species are *A. muscaria*—or fly agaric, named for its purported effectiveness as a household insecticide in the Middle Ages—and A. pantherina or "panther cap," a rarer but more potent species found in Europe and Western Asia.

The *Amanita* species have very little in common with psilocybin-containing "magic mushrooms" (see page 89). Those mushrooms cause a tumult of simultaneous thoughts and feelings, swirling visuals usually recognized as illusory, and a deepening connection to self and body. Fly agaric, however, produces stillness of mind, delusions often mistaken for reality, and a sense of detachment. Psilocybin mushrooms remain far more popular, and *Amanita* mushrooms are not generally considered recreational.

POISON OR SACRED MEDICINE?

Two chemical components account for the effects of *A. muscaria* and *A. pantherina* —muscimol, the key psychoactive compound, and ibotenic acid, which occurs in higher concentrations. A fraction of the ibotenic acid is converted to muscimol in the body; the rest is excreted unchanged in the urine.

An adult dose usually ranges from one to three mushroom caps, but would-be foragers take note: The potency of any given cap depends upon the region and season in which it was harvested. Accidental poisonings, whether from species misidentification or recreational overdose, are common, but fatalities are extremely rare. In fact, few recorded deaths of healthy individuals have ever been linked to *A. muscaria* overdose.

In some very limited contexts, the fly agaric has even been utilized as a food. That's right: If boiled properly to remove all toxins, *A. muscaria* can be safe for the dinner table. In Sanada, a remote town in the Nagano prefecture of Japan, pickled amanita are a traditional treat—albeit an increasingly rare one. During times of economic hardship leading up to World War II, some Italian villages collected, detoxified, and cooked the wild mushrooms to avoid starvation.

These examples are few and far between, however, and casual mycophiles are recommended to stick to more established culinary species—or else be prepared for an unintentional after-dinner vision quest.

AMANITA MUSCARIA INVADES WESTERN CONSCIOUSNESS

Throughout the eighteenth century, strange tales filtered in from travelers who'd visited distant Siberian locales. Whisperings alluded to hardy peoples who herded reindeer in the snowy tundra, ate magical toadstools, and conducted mysterious ceremonies that alternated between raving mania and irresistible lethargy.

The potency of any given cap depends upon the region and season in which it was harvested.

The earliest written report came from Filip Johann von Strahlenberg, a Swedish colonel who was captured by the Russians and lived in Siberia for twelve years as a prisoner of war. In 1730, he published a book that detailed life among the Koryak, a remote Siberian tribe, including their use of the fabled mushroom.

One particular passage describes the Koryak's class divisions in vivid terms. According to von Strahlenberg, those who could afford the prized fly agarics indulged regularly, often selling furs or reindeer to secure them from Russian traders. Others resorted to more creative means: Whenever wealthy people would boil and consume the mushrooms,

> *. . . the poorer sort . . . post themselves, on these occasions, round the huts of the rich, and watch the opportunity of the guests coming down to make water, and then hold a wooden bowl to receive the urine, which they drink off greedily. . . and by this way they also get drunk.*

The division did not always fall between economic classes. In Western Siberia, only the shamans were permitted to eat the mushrooms; other tribe members would consume the shaman's potent urine. In this way, the shaman became both a literal and figurative conduit, channeling the mushroom's divine power for his people.

This seemingly bizarre practice was, in fact, quite practical. In the tundra, ingesting urine served as a way to conserve a precious resource. Indeed, because the human body metabolizes the mushroom's ibotenic acid into the more potent muscimol, the user's urine is said to exceed the strength of fresh mushrooms and even filters out some of the less desirable side effects.

For those who can stomach it, the process can be repeated four or five times before losing its potency altogether. By repeatedly recycling the active compounds, a handful of mushrooms can inebriate many people and extend their altered state for days at a time. If *A. muscaria* is a gift of the gods, as the Siberian shamans believe, it's truly a gift that keeps on giving.

Humans are not alone in eating the fly agarics. Reindeer, too, have a special taste for them. The Sami people in Finland, noticing the animals' predilection for the magical fungus, have been known to collect reindeer urine and drink it for psychoactive effects.

THE FIRST TRIP REPORT

In the century after von Strahlenberg's book was published, a few travelers confirmed his observations, but there were no firsthand accounts to elucidate the mushroom-taker's state of mind. This changed in 1837 when a Polish brigadier named Joseph Kopec published the first personal account of fly agaric intoxication.

While living in a remote region of northeastern Siberia, Kopec became ill and was offered the sacred mushrooms by a local healer. After taking the medicine, Kopec found himself transported to

. . . the most attractive gardens where only pleasure and beauty seemed to rule. Flowers of different colours and shapes and odours appeared before my eyes; a group of most beautiful women dressed in white going to and fro seemed to be occupied with the hospitality of this earthly paradise. As if pleased with my coming, they offered me different fruits, berries, and flowers.

It is difficult, almost impossible, to describe the visions I had in such a long sleep. . . All objects and people that I knew . . . all my games, occupations, actions, one following the other, day after day, year after year, in one word the picture of my whole past become present in my sight.

For Europeans, Kopec's report provided an early glimpse of the obscure fungus and its special status among Far Eastern healers. Later studies and eyewitness accounts illuminated its central role in much of Northern Asia. Far from an isolated phenomenon, the fly agaric was revealed as a vital sacrament among a variety of peoples who lived thousands of miles apart. For some indigenous groups, the mushroom remained their only intoxicant for many centuries—until their Russian neighbors to the south introduced them to alcohol.

THE KORYAK OF KAMCHATKA

The source of most of these stories is Kamchatka, an isolated peninsula hidden in the northeastern corner of Siberia. Kamchatka is a world of fire and ice, its snowy plains dotted with dozens of active volcanoes, hot springs, and geysers.

The traditional Koryak tribes eke out a living along the coasts and in the remote tundra, as they always have. Though they've adapted to the modern world, trading in their traditional reindeer steeds for snowmobiles, their taste for the hallucinogenic mushrooms has persisted through the ages.

Regarding fungi, the approaches of the Russians and the Koryak could not be more different: The Russians collect and eat many varieties of mushrooms, but take care to avoid the poisonous fly agaric. The indigenous people, however, actively seek out the red-and-white mushroom to the exclusion of all others. It is a remarkable demonstration of the degree to which cultural values dictate our attitudes, especially with regard to altered states of consciousness. One man's poison is another man's pleasure.

For the Koyrak, *A. muscaria* is a medicine, mediator of the spirit world, and celebratory intoxicant all in one. Shamans apply it topically to treat injuries and deaden pain. The elderly consume it at night to help them sleep and in the day to promote energy—a clear testament to the spotted beauty's paradoxical effects. Shamans use the fungus to access the spirit world, which enables them to diagnose illnesses, seek the names of newborns, speak with ancestors, and provide hunting advice to the tribe. At seasonal feasts and weddings, everyone consumes the mushroom, often with berry juice.

As a deliriant with remarkable lucidity, a dissociative with tactile and sensual enhancements, and a sedative that grants the user overwhelming strength and endurance, *A. muscaria* is a mushroom of bold contrasts, defined more by its paradoxes than by any consistent effects. Perhaps the oxymoron of "waking dream" describes it best. Moments of terror bleed into fits of ecstasy, and a person may drift from a fevered drumming session into deep sleep without warning.

Nausea, muscle twitches, and profuse sweating and salivation are the most common side effects, but these vary widely with the dose and the person. Vision becomes blurry and coordination is impaired, yet the Koryak say feats of skill and extraordinary strength are common among mushroom-addled tribesmen. The

SOMA AND SANTA CLAUS

Whether because of its quaint fairytale appearance or its bewildering effects, the ancient fly agaric has accumulated a number of myths and legends over the years.

The Rig Veda, an ancient Aryan text dating to 1500 BCE, makes frequent mention of a mysterious sacred substance called "soma." Soma was of great importance to the Aryans, who swept through India and spread its consumption to those they conquered: Of the Rig Veda's 1,028 hymns, 120 are dedicated to this spiritual intoxicant. Yet, we still don't know its identity. The Aryan mushroom cult eventually died out, leaving only the Rig Veda's hymns as tantalizing clues to the soma mystery. Some historians have suggested fly agaric as the most likely candidate, but the evidence is sparse.

In another strange theory that has cropped up in recent years, Santa Claus is merely an anthropomorphized fly agaric spirit. Why do his reindeer fly? They've eaten the sacred mushroom, of course! The more elaborate explanations point to every corner of the modern Santa myth—Santa's gnomish features, his red-and-white suit, the snowy North Pole, and the importance of pine trees and reindeer—as evidence for its long-forgotten Siberian origins. But it all seems rather unlikely. The parallels between *A. muscaria* and the jolly man in the red suit are interesting at first glance, but, like a distant mushroom-induced dream, they fail to materialize into anything substantial.

mushroom's unpredictability has surely contributed to its legendary reputation as a conduit of the gods.

A researcher who spent two years with Siberian tribes described how the men entered fits of ecstasy after taking the sacrament:

> They suddenly sprang raving from their seats and began loudly and wildly calling for drums. . . . And now began an indescribable dancing and singing, a deafening drumming and a wild running about . . . during which the men threw everything about recklessly, until they were completely exhausted. Suddenly they collapsed like dead men and promptly fell into deep sleep.

Another researcher mentions "an inexorable urge to activity," alongside delusions, fits of ecstatic frenzy, prophetic vision, sexual energy, and remarkable strength." Alertness and drowsiness come in waves, like the tide. Dreams are as vivid as reality, and as believable. As with other deliriants, memory is impaired—the user often wakes with an incomplete account of what transpired.

According to novelist Tom Robbins, the fly agaric brings one into contact with that which, "if not actually the godhead, is holistic awareness of the godhead. But it does not do this gently. Instead of slipping one into the cosmic fabric like a silver needle, it drives one in like a wooden stake. And of course, a stake is blunted in the driving."

A GLOBAL FUNGAL NETWORK

A. muscaria is one of the oldest and most widely distributed of all natural sacraments. The Kamchatka peninsula may be the cradle of A. muscaria, but the mysterious fungus has traveled the globe and taken root in other far-flung locations. Applying a bit of imagination, we can view these isolated pockets of mushroom shamanism as part of a broader tradition—local offshoots of a mycelial network whose filaments span the globe and transcend time.

The speckled mushroom colonized ever-more remote locales by entwining itself with human lives, just as its physical form twirled around the roots of pines and birches. Reaching through the fertile medium of human consciousness, the mushroom bears its fruit: not the red and white caps bursting from the loam, but the ineffable visionary experience occasioned in the minds of its followers.

In this view, the specifics of any given mushroom cult fade into the background. What emerges from the varied social fabric is one grand pattern, a symbiotic dance between human-and mushroomkind, which began in prehistory and rolls ever onward into the future. Never entirely forgotten, *A. muscaria* consciousness still blooms in scattered pockets of the world, vibrant and unassuming like mushrooms in a quiet wood.

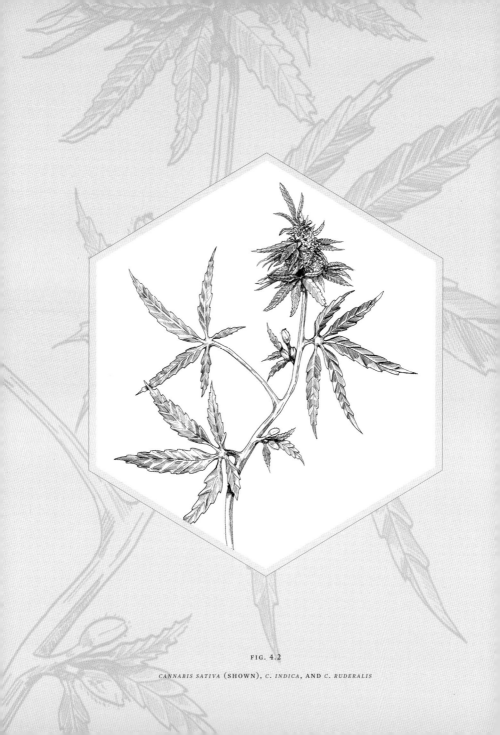

FIG. 4.2

CANNABIS SATIVA (SHOWN), *C. INDICA*, AND *C. RUDERALIS*

CANNABIS

DURATION

3 hours when smoked;
can last 24 hours or more
when eaten

ASSOCIATED WITH *Hindu* sadhus, *artists, musicians, hippies, Rastafari*

ORIGINS AND BACKGROUND

C ANNABIS, MARIJUANA, WEED, POT, GANJA, BHANG, GRASS, BUD— such a profusion of names for one humble plant. The variety of epithets, ranging from the "evil weed" of antidrug propaganda to the holy "bhang" of Hindu tradition, indicates an equally broad spectrum of attitudes toward this truly unusual herb. Both revered and feared, it is perhaps the most misunderstood drug in human history.

Cannabis is the fourth most popular intoxicant in the world, after alcohol, caffeine, and tobacco. Among the safest of all inebriants, cannabis does not cause nearly as many long-term health problems as many other popular substances, nor does it lead to increased violence, risk taking, or criminal behavior. In stark contrast to alcohol and tobacco, cannabis—even according to the DEA—has not been responsible for a single overdose death in recorded history.

Yet, it remains forbidden throughout the majority of the world. In many countries, mere possession can land you in jail. In the twentieth century, the image of cannabis as a stupefying narcotic supplanted the more traditional classifications of as a harmless vice, crucial industrial crop, or divine boon. But cannabis prohibition stands out as an anomaly: Humankind's relationship with the herb has been long and mostly positive. In recent years, the tide has begun to turn toward acceptance, and a groundswell of support has emerged for legalizing cannabis in many corners of the globe.

THE THREE SPECIES OF CANNABIS

The *Cannabis* genus belongs to the small Cannabacae family, which it shares with hackberries and hops, the ingredient that lends bitterness to beer. Though its classification has been debated for centuries, biologists today usually divide the genus into three species: *sativa*, *indica*, and *ruderalis*.

Sativa strains are high in tetrahydrocannabinol, or THC, the compound most responsible for cannabis's psychoactive effects. Indica strains have high levels of cannabidiol, or CBD, a compound that relieves anxiety, protects neurons, and may treat some forms of epilepsy. Sativa-based strains are typically characterized as stimulating and "cerebral," ideal for daytime use, whereas the sedating effects of indica-based strains are better for evenings. The third species, a short-statured Russian variant named *ruderalis*, is rarely marketed because of its inferiority in producing both psychoactive buds and industrial hemp fibers.

For consumers, the distinction is not always useful: Sativa and indica plants cross-pollinate readily, and commercial cannabis strains comprise a full spectrum of hybrids. With evocative names like Strawberry Kush and White Widow, each strain contains a unique profile of cannabinoids, terpenes, and other active components that determine its effects. The plant's complex pharmacology is only just beginning to be understood.

EAT, SMOKE, OR VAPE

After picking a strain, the modern cannabis consumer is confronted with a dizzying selection of formulations. As the legal cannabis market continues to grow, it resembles the burgeoning craft beer movement, with skilled artisans churning out unique flavors and strains by the day. There are magazines featuring cannabis critiques, festivals offering countless samples, and even Cannabis Cup competitions to celebrate the very best products on offer.

The traditional forms are straightforward: There are flowering buds, the iconic green nuggets that most people picture when they think of marijuana.

Hashish, a brown putty made by rolling together the plant's resin glands, offers a higher concentration of active compounds. And then there are edibles—psychoactive foods made from cannabis buds, resin, or even leaves. These range from the milk-based bhang beverage in India to "space cakes" in Amsterdam and everything in between.

The most obvious way to consume it is simply to smoke the bud, but even this has spawned a profusion of gadgets and methods. Perhaps the easiest option is the joint, a rolled-up cannabis cigarette. Others prefer a water pipe, or bong, in which the smoke is drawn through a chamber of water, cooling it before it reaches the smoker's lips.

The most discerning twenty-first-century consumers, however, do not settle for anything as barbaric as setting plant matter on fire. Like many tobacco smokers looking for a healthier alternative, they vaporize instead. Why burn the material to cinders when a precise 350°F (76°C) will do? Vaporizers now come in a plethora of shapes and sizes, ranging from handheld "vape pens" to large machines with removable "whips"—long tubes used for inhaling—or large plastic bags that inflate with vapor.

HASH OIL AND TINCTURES

Modern cannabis culture has not only revolutionized the way the plant is consumed but also the way it is prepared and processed. Hash oil, a purified extract with a very high concentration of psychoactive compounds, has emerged as the latest and hippest cannabis product. Names like *shatter, honeycomb, crumble,* and *pull-and-snap* refer to various textures of hash oil, covering the gamut from honeylike liquids to brittle sheets. Hash oils are consumed in vaporizers or in specialized setups built for "dabbing." After heating a nail or other metal surface with a blowtorch, the user places a "dab" of hash oil on it and inhales the vapors. With up to 90 percent THC content, these extracts pack a powerful punch. By comparison, even buds from the most potent strains rarely surpass 25 percent THC.

If you can eat it and smoke it, why not drink it? As cannabinoids dissolve readily in alcohol, it's only natural that enterprising mixologists have begun crafting cannabis-based tinctures and cocktails. The simplest, sometimes called the "Green Dragon," consists of ground cannabis dissolved in high-proof ethanol, then strained to remove all solids. Most recipes pack a serious wallop: A few droplets on the gums can keep a person high all day.

THE EXPERIENCE

Neither a stimulant nor a depressant, cannabis casts a unique spell on the body and mind. Physically, dry mouth and increased heart rate are typical. The muscles relax and, as just about everyone knows, the eyes redden.

For most people, the draw of cannabis lies in its intriguing mental effects. The main highlights are euphoria and relaxation. Every pleasant sensation becomes more pleasurable—food is more delicious, music becomes exhilarating, and sex is sublime. Some people feel more social under the influence, and cannabis is even being investigated as a treatment for social anxiety.

It's not all good news, however. Some people become anxious and paranoid, even on low doses. Though some negative reactions may be chalked up to a high-

SO MUCH MORE THAN A HIGH

Many parts of the marijuana plant are useful—and not just for getting high. Cannabis has been harvested for its seeds, which once served as a plentiful source of oil for lamplighting, as well as a food among ancient peoples. And the protein-rich seeds are making a comeback—hemp sprouts, hemp milk, hemp oil, and other seed-derived foods are emerging on the modern market.

Through most of history, the plant's prime value was as a source of hemp fibers. An unusually durable stem fiber, hemp has woven its way into a tremendous variety of products, from clothing and footwear to ropes and paper.

During the Colonial era, most European powers depended on hemp to fashion the sails and ropes of their ships. In fact, the word *canvas* derives from cannabis. England's Royal Navy was powered by cannabis—the crop was so essential the British Empire required colonists to grow it to keep their ships freshly stocked. The much later British Invasion of the 1960s may also have been powered by cannabis, but in an altogether different way.

THC strain or poor setting, it's safe to say cannabis doesn't agree with everyone.

Typically presented in pop culture as a "stoning" drug that dumbs down the user, cannabis's real effects are more subtle, especially for those seeking more than a recreational high. Many people cite improved creativity and imagination as a primary motivation for indulging. Freed from its usual routes, one's train of thought traces unexpected paths across the mental landscape. Mundane thoughts and situations become hilarious; truisms and non sequiturs are transformed into nuggets of wisdom.

Although true hallucinations are rare at typical doses, perceptual changes are common. These can range from vibrant scenes imagined behind closed eyes to distortions of time, space, and one's own body. It's not an experience prone to sudden, dramatic epiphanies but rather serene and contemplative states of being. As a substance that frequently occasions a sense of deep connectedness, wonder, and imagination, its classification as a mild psychedelic seems completely appropriate.

CANNABIS AND SPIRITUALITY

For millions of people, cannabis offers an authentic and accessible state of spiritual oneness. Some people incorporate the plant into their personal spiritual practices, without connecting to any particular religious tradition. Others integrate cannabis into personalized variations of religions that do not traditionally embrace the herb, such as Christianity and Judaism. Even atheists have been known to appreciate the nebulous impression of spirituality or occasioned by the plant. But cannabis has not been limited to these sideline roles.

The Hindu god Shiva has long held a particularly close association with the plant. According to legend, Shiva carried cannabis down from the Himalayas to the valleys where people dwelled. Shiva is also considered the Lord of bhang, an umbrella term for cannabis edibles, ranging from savory fritters to small rolled balls of cannabis paste to lassi, a sweet drink based on yogurt or milk.

At annual celebrations held in Shiva's name, bhang lassi flows freely. Sadhus—itinerant holy men who have renounced earthly possessions in favor of prayer and meditation—gather around bonfires, smoking hashish from clay pipes. The sadhus are easily recognized by their yellow robes, long dreadlocked hair, and vibrant face paint. And, of course, by the distinct smell of burnt hashish.

Cannabis has also been a favored inebriant in the Middle East for many centuries. Although most leading Muslim authorities consider it *haram*, or forbidden, hashish remains popular in many Islamic countries today. In fact, the two biggest hashish producers in the world, Afghanistan and Morocco, are Muslim-majority nations. The Sufis, a mystical sect of Muslims who focused on the direct experience of God, embraced cannabis as a sacrament, adopting unorthodox measures that other Muslim sects would shun as haram. Far from unholy, Sufis considered activities such as dancing and cannabis consumption as valid paths to God, if pursued with proper intention.

THE RASTAFARI

Today, the Rastafari are one of the best-known examples of religious cannabis use. Founded by Jamaicans in the 1930s after the coronation of the Ethiopian emperor Haile Selassie, the Rastafari movement accepted the emperor as God incarnate. The Rastafari combine this view with traditional Christian principles, such as the divinity of Jesus, and, of course, the appreciation of cannabis as a sacrament and way of life.

Cannabis is central to the Rastafari way. A Rasta smokes ganja when he needs spiritual counsel from Jah—the Rastafari term for God—and also in communal settings. Rastas come together for "Reasoning" sessions, where adherents smoke the herb from a long-necked water pipe called a *chalice*, meditate together, and debate the best ways to apply their values to everyday life. The Rastafari not only believe that cannabis improves mental clarity and fosters peace, but that its use is divinely sanctioned. They see references to cannabis in the Bible, for instance, the Tree of Life is believed to refer to cannabis and likewise the scripture from Revelation 22:2: "The herb is the healing of nations."

For many people, awareness of the religion came in the form of reggae music. In particular, Bob Marley, the world-famous reggae icon and unabashed cannabis

The Rastafari not only believe that cannabis improves mental clarity and fosters peace, but that its use is divinely sanctioned.

smoker, did much to popularize the movement. Marley's music was deeply affected by his spiritual values, and his seventy-five million sold records—and counting—continue to spread the Rasta way far beyond the borders of Jamaica.

HEALING HERB

For a plant classified by the federal government as having "no currently accepted medical use," cannabis boasts a surprising range of potential medical applications. One may turn out to be chronic pain relief. States with medical marijuana laws show a significant drop in painkiller prescriptions, as well as reductions in hospital admissions relating to opioid abuse and dependence, indicating many people find cannabis preferable to opioids in managing pain. Compared to opioids such as morphine and codeine, cannabis has more agreeable side effects and a lower risk of dependence.

Cannabis is also more effective at treating neuropathic pain (pain caused by nerve damage) where opioids offer little help. In a nation ravaged by opioid addiction, which, according to the CDC, kills more than thirty thousand people per year, an effective painkiller that reduces opioid use should be celebrated as a godsend and prioritized for further study.

The plant can also be used to treat neurological problems, including epilepsy and multiple sclerosis (MS). A study of MS patients showed that cannabis helped reduce their muscle spasms as well as other symptoms of the disease such as overactive bladder and painful sensations. Pure CBD, one of the plant's main cannabinoids, has been shown to reduce seizures, even in the most treatment-resistant forms of epilepsy.

The increased appetite, colloquially known as "the munchies," is utilized by some people to help combat eating disorders. This, combined with its antinausea properties, has made it an ideal substance for both chemotherapy patients and those with AIDS, who often have great difficulty eating.

Cannabis is also a powerful anti-inflammatory. As inflammation is such a common component in many diseases, cannabis may have beneficial effects on a wide range of conditions including Crohn's disease, atherosclerosis, rheumatoid arthritis, inflammation associated with certain cancers, and—somewhat surprisingly, for a substance most often smoked—asthma.

The list continues. By reducing internal eye pressure, cannabis may prove useful in treating glaucoma. And early research suggests THC and other cannabinoids can target brain cancer cells, shrinking tumors in mice.

The herb is good for more than just bodily complaints. Its effects on consciousness have found favor among people with PTSD, and its anxiety-reducing effects are famous. Some people claim a mood-stabilizing effect, and early research indicates it may help relieve stress-related depression.

HEALTH PROBLEMS

Cannabis is not a miracle cure, however. Most of its medical benefits remain anecdotal or speculative, and it does have real side effects. Some people complain of dizziness, fatigue, vomiting, and even hallucinations. Long-term use, though far safer than common drugs like tobacco and alcohol, has its share of problems. True to the "stoner" stereotype, chronic heavy users have a higher risk of depression, tiredness, and a general lack of motivation.

Formulations with THC can negatively affect memory and thought processes, producing a mental fog that only abstinence can lift. Though claims that it makes people crazy are vastly exaggerated, cannabis can induce psychosis in people predisposed to schizophrenia and may hasten the onset of the disease.

Although cannabis smoke includes many of the same toxins and carcinogens as tobacco smoke, no definitive link between moderate smoking and lung cancer has been discovered. Though there may be a limited correlation, it's clear any lung damage from cannabis pales in comparison to that of tobacco.

These results puzzled researchers and medical experts, who suggest that cannabis smoke may contain antioxidant and other protective components that counteract the harmful effects of the carcinogens. That's not to say smoking cannabis is perfectly safe on the lungs—heavy smokers may experience reduced breathing capacity and lung inflammation that can cause asthma-like symptoms after many years. Vaporizing greatly reduces these risks.

The twentieth century was not kind to cannabis, but it's finally getting its day in the sun. Many countries in Latin America and Europe have decriminalized the possession of small amounts, including Portugal, Spain, Colombia, Ecuador, Mexico, Peru, and Chile. Jamaica, home of the Rastafari, finally decriminalized possession in 2015. Uruguay, recognizing that prohibition fostered a black market far more toxic than the plant itself, legalized it altogether in 2014—the first country to do so. In the Netherlands, "coffeeshops" have been serving up bud since the 1970s, though it remains technically illegal.

Even Americans are coming around. Legalization is now supported by a majority of Americans and has become something of a rallying cry for many political candidates—a stance that would have meant political suicide not long ago. Pot, the enduring symbol of the counterculture, is officially mainstream.

People in a majority of all states now have legal access to medical marijuana. Nine states and the District of Columbia (and counting) have fully legalized the plant, including California—the sixth largest economy in the world. Altogether, more than seventy million Americans enjoy access to legal recreational cannabis.

While there has been progress, the US remains in a state of transition. The federal government has not moved from the position of steadfast prohibition. Cannabis businesses have been forced to deal in cash because national banks, fearful of repercussions from the federal government, refused their business. Until the national laws change, neither business owners nor consumers have any guarantee the feds won't come knocking, as they have in countless dispensary and home raids in the past.

Nevertheless, prohibition is crumbling. With each state that legalizes, the federal government's position becomes increasingly untenable. Attitudes and laws are changing, not just in the United States but around the world.

Most of its medical benefits remain anecdotal or speculative, and it does have real side effects.

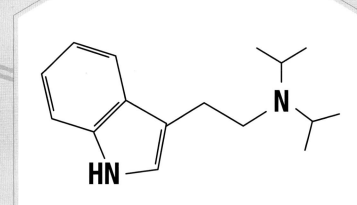

FIG. 4.3

N,N-DIISOPROPYLTRYPTAMINE

DIPT

FAMOUS FOR *auditory distortions*

ORIGINS AND BACKGROUND

IF THERE IS ONE SENSE ASSOCIATED WITH THE PSYCHEDELIC experience, it is sight. Assessing a new compound, trippers rate its "visuals" the way wine aficionados speak of the nose or finish of a favored vintage. Whether it's shifting, drifting, morphing, or distorting, something is happening visually or else you got a dud. To be sure, psychedelics are known to affect other senses—especially touch and hearing—but, for many people, "seeing things" is the bread and butter of tripping.

Now imagine a psychedelic substance that forgoes visual effects altogether. When chemists Alexander Shulgin and Michael Carter first introduced the world to DiPT in a 1980 research paper, their description was at first unremarkable: "At no time was sensory distortion in the visual field observed" in human subjects.

But DiPT had one characteristic that made it stand out from all other psychoactive substances: It created "an unusual disturbance in the integrity of the auditory processes." In other words, Shulgin and his colleague had found an auditory hallucinogen. Under the influence of DiPT, everything sounded lower in pitch. Voices deepened, guitars clanged like giant gongs, and music lost all harmony.

Since those early days—and especially since Shulgin's 1997 publication *TiHKAL (Tryptamines I Have Known and Loved)*, in which he laid out the substance's effects as well as steps for its chemical synthesis—DiPT's fame as the sound-warping substance has only grown. Among musicians, novelty seekers, and those curious about the brain's sound-processing abilities, no substance is more beguiling.

THE EXPERIENCE

DiPT can be eaten, vaporized, or insufflated (sniffed). The latter is said to be incredibly painful, so, although the substance both smells and tastes disgusting, most users opt to swallow it. With this method, the main experience lasts between 8 and 12 hours, though the auditory effects can linger for a full 36 hours.

The first hour or two can be physically uncomfortable. The energy rush has been likened to the onset of MDMA, and the light-headedness and shortened attention span are common to many stimulants and psychedelics. The bloating, nausea, and sometimes-painful inner-ear pressure, however, read more like the side effects list from a pharmaceutical ad.

Then, several hours in—just when the explorer is ready to write off the substance's hype as a cruel hoax—the audio effects begin in earnest. Mercifully, the indigestion often subsides around the same time.

The first alert often comes in the form of an unmistakable shift in one's speaking voice—"Is that really what I sound like?" In Shulgin's *TiHKAL*, an anonymous tester describes this bizarre warping:

The voices of people were extremely distorted—males sounded like frogs—children sounded like they were talking through synthesizers to imitate outer space people in science fiction movies.

But DiPT is not merely a helium balloon in reverse, deepening voices instead of transforming them into cartoonish squeaks. All sounds are affected, especially those with a well-defined pitch. One amateur musician offers a detailed description:

> Lower tones were distinctly embellished, sounding warmer, fuller, and layered with harmonic tones, while higher tones seemed to be relatively unaffected . . . The primary tone was intact, but there were several lower harmonic and melodic tones resonating at the same time.

Like a warbled tape deck, not all sounds are affected equally. While low tones tend to get even lower, high pitches instead burst with chirping and stretching sounds: "Inhaling, it sounds like high-pitched wire tension noises are happening within that breath."

But how does it affect music? The results are in, and they're not pretty. "Piano sounds like a bar-room disaster," one early tester told Shulgin.

A more recent experimenter watched a video of a symphony orchestra: "Predictably enough, it sounded like nobody had practiced and the conductor was drunk and insane." Clearly, this is not the substance to take before your favorite band goes on stage.

Shulgin explained why everything sounds dissonant, even an unaccompanied solo instrument: "You play an oboe . . . and it no longer sounds like an oboe because all the harmonics are out of pitch with one another, no longer harmonically related." The delicate tonal balance is destroyed. What's left is dreck: "It's just ugly music."

Or perhaps not. Others have described profound sonic experiences with the drug. According to some, the secret is choosing music that's already dissonant— it can hardly go out of tune if it's not in tune to begin with. A bit of garage punk or minimalist techno, for instance, can transform into something fresh without becoming unlistenable in the process.

The secret is choosing music that's already dissonant—it can hardly go out of tune if it's not in tune to begin with.

It's not always "an aural toy box of ear-tickling proportions," as one psychonaut put it. The compound's disconcerting effects on sound are often accompanied by physical sensations in the ear, as though plugged up by wax. DiPT users sometimes feel the need to yawn, as though ascending in an airplane, but find no relief.

This inner ear pressure increases with the dose and can be painful. Tinnitus—a sometimes disturbingly loud ringing, most noticeable in a silent environment—is also common. Both symptoms can last for days, or even weeks, afterward, especially with very high doses. Whether these sensations are related to DiPT's pitch-bending effect remains unknown.

A FRESH TAKE ON AN OLD TUNE

Our ability to recognize sounds depends greatly on its tonal color, or timbre. Timbre, in turn, depends on a sound's full harmonic spectrum—the gamut of "overtones" produced along with the fundamental note. Our ears and brains have evolved to parse these sonic signatures, and are capable of identifying a dizzying variety of sounds almost instantly. You can easily tell a trombone from a violin, even if they're playing the same note.

That's why the DiPT experience is so bewildering: By unpredictably shifting all pitches, it messes with our ability to identify their sources. On DiPT, a guitar doesn't simply become a bass guitar; it transforms into a dissonant glockenspiel. Even drums are unrecognizable, clanging like steel pipes in an echo chamber.

As a result, a song you've heard a hundred times can sound utterly foreign. Upon putting on one of her favorite electronic tracks, one user was

> . . . nearly moved to tears by what I heard . . . [it was] one of the most amazing drug effects I have ever encountered or probably ever will encounter: the ability to re-experience something beloved as completely new again . . . It is something I expect to remember vividly for a very, very long time.

MORE THAN A SOUND EFFECT?

Reading through the reports, you might get the impression that DiPT is purely auditory—a simple digital-effects box contained in a white powder. At low to moderate doses, that may be so.

But those who venture deeper have discovered much more, and they dispute the compound's reputation as a one-trick pony. In particular, several explorers cite a new appreciation for the way sounds guide our perception of the world around us and our ability to navigate it. After experiencing DiPT, one person writes, "I listen much more closely to all sounds around me, and actually appreciate them for what they are instead of treating them as background noise."

Perhaps most surprising are the visual effects of this supposedly audio-only substance. With high enough doses—*and don't try this at home, kids*—the most intrepid explorers have found that DiPT does indeed produce visionary distortions. These range from bursts of light behind closed eyes to full-blown hallucinations:

> *I stepped outside and looked at the sky in awe . . . The clouds were turning into balls of fire that resembled meteors and they started falling from the sky. It was the end of a most incredible night.*

These doses are not for the faint of heart. At this level, the audio distortions become overwhelming and it is nearly impossible to maintain a conversation. Those looking for visual effects should stick with more traditional psychedelics.

Such a unique chemical seems ripe for psychological research. As three researchers note, DiPT warrants

> . . . *further investigation from those interested in the neurology of sound, music, and verbal language processing. For example, it would be fascinating to know the effects of this substance on perceptions of tonal languages such as Chinese, Huichol, or Dogon; would it alter the words perceived as being spoken?*

Shulgin, the molecule's original discoverer, suggested several avenues of research. He asked, "Is there an area in the brain that is uniquely dedicated to the pitch of sound?" With DiPT, we might be able to find out. He recommended using a modified version of the molecule as a tracer, to follow its path through the human brain. Where does it collect most densely? Which neural regions are most affected?

Never one to stop asking questions, Shulgin considered some more imaginative possibilities: "What would be the scan of its distribution in a tone-deaf subject? What would be its effect on a schizophrenic subject who is hearing the voice of God?"

Studying the way DiPT works its magic may reveal more about how the brain interprets sounds and music. We know serotonin is linked to the inner ear and the vestibular system; but how? The fact that DiPT affects both the physical ear and the brain's auditory processing hints at a complex multimodal effect.

As Shulgin also noted, we can use DiPT as a baseline to develop other auditory compounds. Simple tweaks could result in several different chemicals, which "might well have even more remarkable and specific properties. If you don't look, you won't find."

The unfortunate news is that we aren't looking. With the exception of illicit psychonauts, DiPT research has been all but shelved since Shulgin's first investigations. Perhaps one day, the famed auditory hallucinogen will help scientists shed light on how we perceive sounds and music.

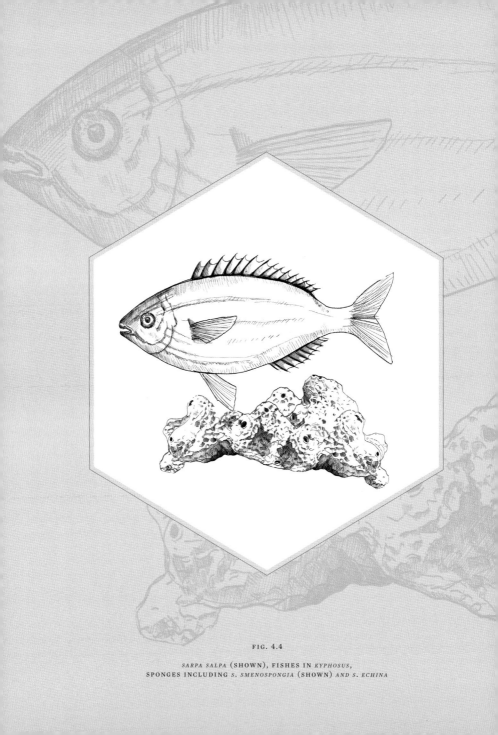

FIG. 4.4

SARPA SALPA (SHOWN), FISHES IN *KYPHOSUS*,
SPONGES INCLUDING *S. SMENOSPONGIA* (SHOWN) AND *S. ECHINA*

DISCOVERED

Hallucinogenic fish known
since ancient times;
psychedelic sponges first
confirmed in 2014

FISH AND
SEA SPONGES

DURATION

Fish intoxication: up to
36 hours; 5-Bromo-DMT
from sponges: 90 minutes,
or less time when smoked

NATIVE TO *fish—coastal waters off Africa, Australia, and in the Mediterranean; sponges—the Caribbean*

ORIGINS AND BACKGROUND

F OR MOST PEOPLE, THE PHRASE "NATURAL PSYCHEDELIC" brings to mind a variety of plants, ranging from ayahuasca vines to peyote cacti, and a handful of psychoactive fungi. But all of these are land-based species. Often overlooked is that vast and enigmatic world that exists alongside ours yet remains alien to us—the oceans. Water covers 71 percent of our planet's surface, but the biochemistry of sea creatures remains relatively unexplored. We have ample evidence of life's ingenuity in conjuring intoxicating chemicals on land—what molecular treasure might lie in the murky depths of the sea?

Our current knowledge provides two fascinating examples of sea organisms containing visionary chemicals. First, a surprising number of fish species have been known to cause *ichthyoallyeinotoxism*, or hallucinogenic fish inebriation. This is distinguished from other, less trippy varieties of fish poisoning by the presence of vivid auditory and visual hallucinations that can last for several days. In some cultures, especially among islanders in Polynesia and the Indian Ocean, there is an ongoing tradition of intentional fish intoxication. But for the casual seafood enthusiast, such "trips"—complete with nausea, dizziness, and disturbing nightmares—are accidental and decidedly unpleasant.

The second example is more recent and has absolutely no history of ritual use by humans—at least not yet. Among the humble sea sponges, there are species that produce molecules seen nowhere else in nature—namely, 5-Bromo-DMT, which has been identified as a likely psychedelic.

The "bromo" refers to bromine. Because bromine is very rare in the earth's crust, it almost never appears in the chemistry of land-based organisms. But in the ocean, bromine is much more common, and at least a handful of sea sponges have incorporated it into their internal molecular factories. Sponges, it turns out, are the clandestine chemists of the ocean floor and having churned out unusual compounds for millennia without attracting notice, very successful ones at that.

SARPA SALPA AND OTHER "DREAM FISH"

Among all fish species known to cause hallucinations, the best known is the salema porgy, a sea bream native to coastal waters off Africa, Hawaii, and Australia, as well as the Mediterranean Sea. Boasting the melodious Latin name *Sarpa salpa*, the salema porgy has become famous as both a poison and an intoxicant. Its brilliant golden stripes are immediately recognizable, but mean different things to different people: In Tunisia, France, and Israel, the salema porgy is served like any other fish, while in Italy and Spain, it's considered inedible.

The salema porgy may be the most famous "dream fish," but it is far from the only one. Various species of mullet, grouper, sea chub, rabbitfish, and goatfish have all been known to induce hallucinations. Risk of intoxication increases greatly when the head is eaten—it seems the relevant chemicals are most concentrated in the fish's brain.

For locals of many tropical islands, the danger of intoxication is not common or severe enough to avoid these species altogether. But because of their visionary characteristics, the fish inspire evocative names wherever they are found—the rabbitfish *Siganus spinus* is known on the island of Réunion as "the fish that inebriates," the yellowstripe goatfish is known in Hawaii as "weke pahulu" after the trickster god of nightmares, and the Arabic name for the sea bream *Sarpa salpa* translates to "the fish that makes dreams."

People report a variety of symptoms, but frightening nightmares and hallucinations, poor coordination, blurry vision, disorientation, and impaired memory are common. Tightness in the chest is another frequent complaint. Many patients, blindsided by the unexpected onset of such disturbing symptoms, believe they are dying and start to panic. The nature of the experience appears inconsistent with classical psychedelics, such as LSD or psilocybin, and may point instead to a deliriant active compound.

In spite of its unpleasantness, "poisoning" events are not always accidental. Ancient Romans throughout the Mediterranean were said to consume the fish to embark on extreme mental voyages. Surely, fish tripping marks one of the most unusual of the Roman Empire's many discoveries and strange vices.

Polynesian islanders once incorporated the fish into visionary ceremonies. The details have been lost to time, but some natives still cook up known hallucinogenic fish when they feel like kicking back and, well, hallucinating. Those

THE MYSTERY OF
DREAM FISH CHEMISTRY

What's the trippy ingredient that makes some fish hallucinogenic? No one knows. Although episodes of hallucinogenic fish poisoning are fairly well documented, they're not at all well understood. Studies are confounded by the phenomenon's sporadic nature. Most of the time, fish from affected species are safe to eat, but in some specimens and some seasons—especially spring and summer—the danger increases. Symptoms and duration vary, and it's not always easy to tell when someone has suffered ichthyoallyeinotoxism rather than another foodborne illness.

Further complicating matters, hallucinogenic poisonings may be caused by many different compounds, which may vary by species. And then there's the question of origin—do these fish produce psychedelic compounds on their own, or, as some scientists have speculated, do they acquire them from microbes in their diet? Most dream fish are herbivores; the intense but inconsistent effects may derive from a form of plankton called *dinoflagellates*, from plants known as seagrasses, or from seaweeds in the genus *Caulerpa*.

who enjoy this briny variety of intoxication make no attempt to remove the fish heads, instead mixing them right into their stews to increase their potency.

In a 1960 issue of *National Geographic*, on a visit to Norfolk Island off the coast of Australia, photographer Joe Roberts sampled the local dream fish. He reported visions of a futuristic nature: "I saw a new kind of car, steered with a stick like a plane. And then I was taking pictures of a monument to mark man's first trip into space." His zoologist colleague also tried the dish—"tasty, but strong-flavored, like mackerel"—and reported bizarre dreams.

Most accounts are not so positive, perhaps because they come from medical reports, which by their nature are limited to adverse reactions. In one case, a middle-aged man vacationing in the French Riviera enjoyed baked sea bream for dinner, which turned out to be a toxic specimen of *Sarpa salpa*.

Within hours he began experiencing nausea, fatigue, and muscle weakness. When his symptoms continued through the following day, he opted to end his vacation early and head home. But while driving, the man's symptoms took a turn for the worse: his vision blurred, and he began to see "aggressive and screaming animals" wherever he looked. As the case report nonchalantly states, the man had to pull over and call an ambulance because "he was seeing giant arthropods around his car." Medical examination discovered no physical problems—just lingering delirium, which resolved 36 hours after his ill-fated dinner. Upon recovering, he had no memory of the terrifying hallucinations.

SPONGES AND DMT OF THE SEA

Psychedelic sponges are, if possible, even more mystifying than the dream fish. Sponges are a bit trippy to begin with—although classified as animals, they have no circulatory systems, digestive organs, or nerves. Nor do they have any means of moving around. Indeed, they have no organs or tissues at all; sponges are essentially porous, cylindrical filters, gathering nutrients from water passing through their elaborate cellular networks and from photosynthetic microorganisms residing upon and within them.

In 1997, the celebrated psychedelic chemist Alexander Shulgin alluded to potentially psychedelic alkaloids in sponges. He noted that *Smenospongia aurea*, a small yellow reef sponge native to the Gulf of Mexico and the Caribbean, contains 5-Bromo-DMT, which, Shulgin posited, just might be active when smoked. If so, that would make 5-Bromo-DMT the ocean's first known contribution to the growing list of natural psychedelics. In typical Shulgin fashion, he then joked about starting a rumor, "that all the hippies of the San Francisco Bay Area were heading to the Caribbean with packets of Zig-Zag papers, to hit the sponge trade with a psychedelic fervor."

About fifteen years later, Shulgin's suspicions appeared to be confirmed by a solitary sponge smoker. The source, an anonymous chemist who seems to be the first person to ingest a psychedelic of marine origin, wrote a letter to Hamilton Morris, a journalist covering the psychoactive drug beat for *Vice News*. In the letter, he describes a simpler and more economical way to synthesize 5-Bromo-DMT in the lab than to extract it from nature—good news for the sponges and for aspiring consciousness explorers with no access to exotic underwater critters. More important, the chemist provided the long-awaited confirmation that 5-Bromo-DMT *is* active when smoked and offered his own enlightening firsthand reports.

Taken orally, the effect on consciousness was, "indistinct and short-lived." Perhaps, like its chemical cousin, DMT, it is rapidly metabolized by the body's enzymes and rendered inactive when taken this way.

Smoking the substance produced far more intriguing results; 5-Bromo-DMT was, "definitely psychedelic with a strong tactile side."

> *I closed my eyes and found myself drifting through the ocean on an ice floe shaped like a puzzle piece. . . . Very light and nonaggressive, nonnauseating. Drugs such as this are aptly described as 'serenic.'*

Later, after smoking 50 milligrams of the undersea inebriant:

Upon taking the last large hit I was enveloped by a sensation of heaviness, which was paradoxically light and spacious. . . . My head and hands felt as though they could detach and float away from my body. . . . At another point I felt as though gravity had changed in a similar manner that one would experience while submerged in water . . .

MORE TO DISCOVER

There are an estimated 8.7 million species in the world, one-fourth of which are thought to reside in the oceans. We are still only beginning to understand the complex ecosystems of those unplumbed depths. And when it comes to molecular cocktails and defense toxins, perfected by many thousands of aquatic species over millions of years, we've barely scratched the surface—so to speak.

In particular, marine invertebrates provide an abundance of compounds that resemble serotonin and dopamine—chemical messengers fundamental to human consciousness and intimately involved in mental illnesses such as depression, anxiety, and addiction. Yet in spite of their potential as medicines and entheogens, these undersea chemicals remain almost completely unexplored. Novel psychoactive substances may hide in the darkness of the ocean's deepest corners or perhaps in plain sight among microbes and algae on shallow-water reefs. What chemical clues lie waiting to be discovered?

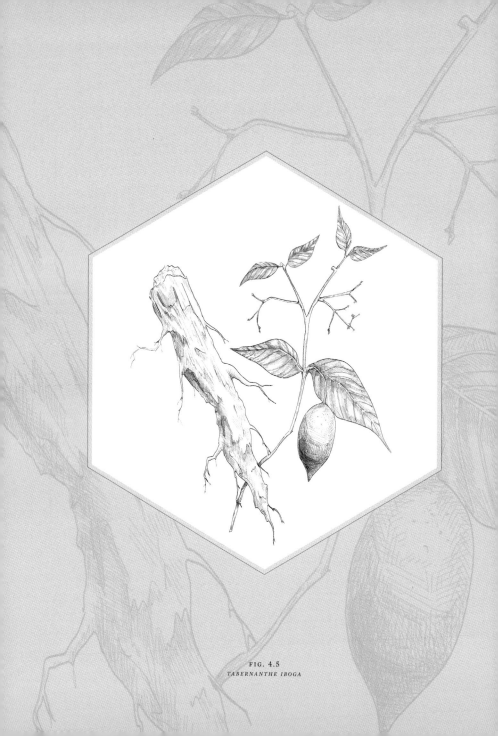

FIG. 4.5
TABERNANTHE IBOGA

KNOWN AS *the sacrament of the Bwiti religion; a potential treatment for addiction*

KEY COMPOUND *ibogaine*

ORIGINS AND BACKGROUND

IN GABON, A SMALL COUNTRY ON THE WESTERN COAST OF CENTRAL AFRICA, iboga is easy to find—the shrub grows in the wild, and a powder made from its roots serves as the sacrament and very foundation of the popular Bwiti religion. It can also be found in a number of luxurious, if unorthodox, detox centers in various parts of the world, including Mexico, Costa Rica, the Netherlands, New Zealand, and even Canada. According to its many believers, iboga stops withdrawal completely and offers a fresh start to people struggling with addiction. But, in the United States and a handful of other countries, iboga and its chief active compound, ibogaine, are banned and very difficult to find on the black market due to their lack of recreational appeal. Advocates for the plant's addiction-fighting qualities are eager to change that, but scientific studies have been slow in coming.

Iboga is a rainforest shrub growing to about 6 feet (1.8 m) in height, with white and pink flowers and distinctive orange fruits. For spiritual ceremonies and drug treatment centers, however, the roots are the main attraction. They contain a mix of many alkaloids, but the strangest and best known is ibogaine. Ibogaine's effects on the brain and body are complex: Like psilocybin and LSD, with which it shares a common structure, it shows activity at serotonin receptors, which likely explains its more visionary qualities. Unlike those molecules, however, ibogaine also has strong activity at several other receptor types, including those utilized by ketamine and salvia to produce their dissociative, mind-bending effects. It's unclear how exactly these receptors elicit ibogaine's putative anti-addictive properties.

No one knows exactly how long iboga has featured as a spiritual medicine among indigenous peoples in western Central Africa. In the late nineteenth century, some of the native Bantu peoples, facing persecution from French missionaries, fled to the forests. There, they encountered the Babongo, a Pygmy tribe with secret knowledge of a powerful root, which they shared with the Bantu visitors. Thus, the Bwiti religion was born, or perhaps remade: a heavily ancestor-focused tradition that featured iboga as its sacrament in various ceremonies and rites of passage.

Bwiti has evolved into numerous sects and spread from Gabon into neighboring countries. The Bantu did not escape the missionaries completely: Many modern Bwiti traditions combine their roots of animism, iboga journeying, and ancestor worship with elements of Catholicism. Other groups have steadfastly resisted outside influences and continue to practice the religion as their forebears learned it more than a century ago. The Catholic Church has disavowed the syncretic, Christianized form of Bwiti, but the religion is here to stay: It's one of the three official religions in Gabon, and in 2000, the country's Council of Ministers declared iboga a national treasure.

GATEWAY TO THE ANCESTORS

The most intense ceremonies of the Bantu—using the highest doses of iboga—are reserved for boys entering manhood. The initiates are covered head to toe in white paint with occasional dark splashes and robed in white cloth. They consume large amounts of the root bark over the course of several days. When they enter an almost comatose state, they are taken to a secluded temple to complete their journey. There they speak to their ancestors, who confer directly with the gods.

When the nganga is satisfied that the boys have seen Bwiti—the realm we all reach upon our deaths and which is available to the living only through the power of iboga—the initiation is complete. The boys have become *baanzi*, those who know the other world. Knowledge of Bwiti is sacred and lifelong—having seen the far shores of reality, a baanzi can, at any time, reconnect with his ancestors by consuming iboga.

Iboga is central to the Bwiti way of life. It is used by the Bantu peoples to connect with the spiritual realm, diagnose the sick, and to honor—and even meet—their ancestors. In each Bantu community, the spiritual leader and expert herbalist, known as the *nganga*, leads the ceremonies. These elaborate rituals, which often go on for several days, usually incorporate singing, dancing, and musicians playing drums, harps, and rattles.

THE EXPERIENCE

In small doses, ibogaine has a stimulant effect. West African tribes have utilized the plant in sub-psychedelic doses to stay alert for long journeys and hunting expeditions.

A large dose, however, provides a profound psychedelic journey. The first sign is a loud, oscillating tone that pervades the user's hearing. Some find the sound distracting or unpleasant, but, in a traditional setting, Bwiti ceremonial music frequently drowns it out.

A condition known as ataxia quickly sets in: the limbs become rubbery, and the subject cannot stand or walk steadily. The lack of coordination is heightened by an intense, motion-sensitive feeling of nausea. Even small movements, such as turning one's head, are likely to cause vomiting. Ibogaine also produces strong photosensitivity, so light becomes painful to bear. With such intense physical side effects, it's easy to see why users usually lie down in the dark, trying to remain completely still—and also why ibogaine has never caught on as a recreational psychedelic.

The experience is generally split into two phases. The visionary state, lasting from 3 to 6 hours, consists of vivid waking dreams, memories, and imagined scenes. Like dreams, they appear laden with surreal and often symbolic content. People often describe them as fast-moving films or slideshows from one's past, including formative childhood scenes rendered in hyper-realistic detail.

Although neither Bwiti practitioners nor drug treatment centers focus on this aspect, extreme distortions of body image are also common during the visual stage. According to one user on Erowid, the online library of drug information:

Senses of light-weightedness and heavy-weightedness alternated. Another characteristic sensation can only be described as falling inwards through my own body. While seated, my feet could appear paradoxically close to my pelvis, or my neck could appear surprisingly long.

The subject may also encounter one or more "spirits" during this time. According to Bwiti tradition, these spirits help guide the initiate to the realm of the ancestors, but such encounters are not limited to the Bwiti ceremonial context. One user, after describing a harrowing session of "skulls rolling, death, trees in blossom, all manner of bestial vision," writes that finally,

. . . the unintelligible brutality of these visions began to clear, and I perceived myself suspended in some sort of celestial chapel, the pillars of such energy as can only be seen on a huge scale, and bedecked by stars. I was introduced . . . to my 'pilots' and they reassured me that I was being guided and that in fact I have never been alone . . . .

The second phase is introspective. Much longer and less visual than the first, this stage often consists of a "life review" resulting in valuable insights. These realizations are often related to the imagery from the first few hours.

Between the vividly reimagined life scenes and honest, searing evaluations that come afterward, seekers are granted a unique opportunity for personal epiphanies. Perhaps it is this change in perspective combined with the compound's withdrawal-stopping effects that allow some people with addiction to walk away truly changed. This phase can last from 8 to 20 hours, and residual stimulation lasts for days, or even weeks afterward.

For followers of Bwiti, it's the gateway to the spiritual plane; for many people addicted to opioids, it means hope. Today it rivals ayahuasca as an intriguing, if little understood, therapeutic treatment among those with means. But how did an African sacrament become co-opted by the international addiction treatment community?

Howard Lotsof was nineteen and addicted to heroin when he discovered ibogaine. He was in the Lower East Side of Manhattan, far from the Bwiti elders of Gabon, when he first encountered the substance as an obscure recreational drug. He was chasing a high, but wound up with a profound healing experience. Lotsof was shocked: After a grueling 36-hour experience, his cravings for heroin had disappeared. When he gave ibogaine to seven of his friends—all addicted to heroin—five of them kicked the habit.

Realizing he'd hit upon something revolutionary, Lotsof became a tireless advocate for ibogaine research. More than anyone else, this recovered heroin addict brought ibogaine to the attention of the Western world. Until his death in 2010, he published papers, patented ibogaine addiction treatments, and petitioned both governments and pharmaceutical companies to support further research.

After the FDA banned ibogaine in 1967, Lotsof moved to the Netherlands and began the first major ibogaine addiction study. Two-thirds of the 30 subjects treated in that study quit using drugs and remained clean for months and, in some cases, years afterward. This was remarkable—with conventional treatments, 90 percent of opioid-dependent people relapse within the first year.

In the late 1980s and early 1990s, a handful of studies with animal models found that ibogaine reduced consumption of morphine, cocaine, and alcohol in substance-dependent rats and mice. A few studies have since extended these results to humans with addiction, and thousands of cases of ibogaine-assisted withdrawal treatment have been documented, but data on long-term results are still lacking.

Thousands of cases of ibogaine-assisted withdrawal treatment have been documented.

The limited evidence was enough to convince the National Institute on Drug Abuse to undertake an ibogaine investigation project in 1991. Just four years later, in the wake of a fatality at a Dutch heroin rehabilitation clinic in which ibogaine was implicated, the NIDA decided to discontinue the project. The pharmaceutical industry has also ignored this potential avenue of research, and why wouldn't they? There's little money to be made in a substance that helps cure addiction in just one or two doses.

BEYOND ADDICTION

Some psychiatrists had already adopted ibogaine as a useful substance in psychotherapy before hearing of Lotsof's research, but none had discovered its potential as an addiction treatment. For these therapists, ibogaine served a more traditional therapeutic role—uncovering repressed memories, shining new light on deeply held pain and trauma, and providing a new perspective on the subject's life and relationships.

When Howard Lotsof met with Leo Zeff, a therapist who had incorporated ibogaine, LSD, and other psychedelics into his practice, and told him about its effectiveness as an addiction treatment, Zeff reexamined his old files. Of all the patients to whom he'd administered ibogaine, only three had had substance abuse problems. All three had quit their habits after the ibogoaine session.

"Of everything we tried," Zeff told Lotsof, "ibogaine achieved the most profound personal transformation of the patient—which after all is the goal and purpose of psychiatry. When it worked, the therapist was just a bystander."

In the last thirty years, there have been about twenty reported deaths relating to ibogaine, but most of them appeared to have complicating factors. In many cases, these deaths resulted from unsafe drug combinations, including opioids; in others, the cause was a preexisting medical condition—particularly heart disease—or complications related to substance withdrawal.

Ibogaine does have real risks and must be administered carefully, especially to drug-addicted individuals. In addition to eliminating opioid withdrawal symptoms, ibogaine also resets a person's tolerance. A treatment subject who relapses after an ibogaine session and ingests the usual amount is likely to overdose. In a clinical setting, these risks can be reduced by prescreening subjects for health conditions, such as heart problems, providing proper support and aftercare, and establishing strict measures to avoid the smuggling of drugs into the treatment center.

For now, ibogaine remains prohibited in the United States, though underground and offshore clinics continue to provide ibogaine therapy to well-connected people. In the near future, it's likely that both international and black market ibogaine clinics will continue welcoming streams of people desperate for a second chance. Perhaps someday, if growing evidence confirms what its believers have been claiming for decades, this unassuming shrub from the shady undergrowth of the African rainforest will finally have its day in the sun.

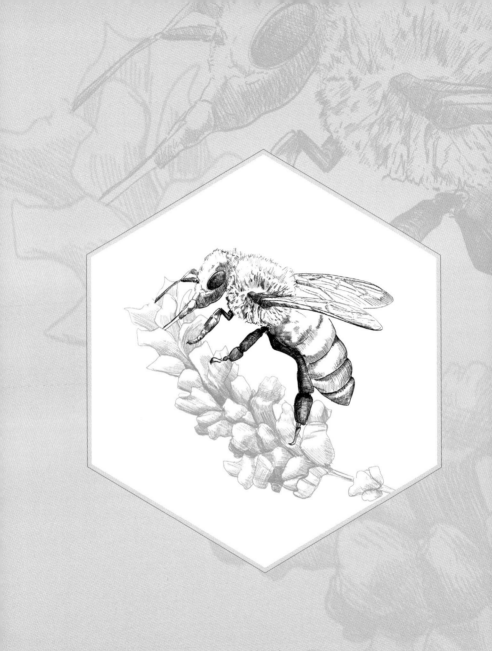

FIG. 4.6
APIS DORSATA LABORIOSA,
OR HIMALAYAN GIANT HONEYBEE

MAD HONEY

ASSOCIATED WITH *the nectar of toxic species of rhododendrons, azaleas, and mountain laurel*

HARVESTED IN *Turkey and Nepal*

ORIGINS AND BACKGROUND

PROBABLY THE LAST THING YOU EXPECT when savoring a spoonful of honey is to wind up in the hospital with dizziness, tingling extremities, and an altered state of mind. But if that golden syrup is "mad honey"—or *deli bal* in Turkish—that's a very real risk and, for its connoisseurs, the whole point of consuming it. Mad honey is produced only in regions where particular species of rhododendron, azalea, and mountain laurel grow rampant, especially in the Himalayan cliffs of central Asia and along the southern shores of the Black Sea in Turkey. These species contain grayanotoxins, a group of poisonous chemicals that affect the central nervous system.

With a history as both biological weapon and prized inebriant, the honey's "mad" moniker is well earned. The nectar's toxins have no effect on bees, but, for humans, the resulting honey is incredibly potent.

THE EXPERIENCE

One spoonful of mad honey is enough to cause noticeable mental and bodily effects, including a mental high, sensations of movement, and spatial disorientation. Higher doses lead to convulsions, hallucinations, vomiting, and problems with breathing and circulation.

Honey intoxication causes a handful of hospital visits every year and in very rare instances can be fatal. In small amounts, however, the honey is relatively safe, and for centuries people have enjoyed the subtle changes in consciousness it provides. Clearly, this is one sweet that demands moderation.

THE HONEY TRAP

More than once, mad honey has swayed the course of history. In 401 BCE, the Athenian general Xenophon led an army of ten thousand back to their Greek homeland after waging war against Persia. Camped along the shores of the Black Sea in today's northeastern Turkey, the army plundered local beehives and gorged themselves on honey, only to find themselves incapacitated with dizziness, diarrhea, and nausea for several days.

More than three centuries later, Roman troops led by General Pompey suffered a similar fate while pursuing a Persian army through the same region. This time it was no accident: The Persians, familiar with the dangers of mad honey, laid out pots of the sweet stuff for the Romans to find. After gobbling down the honey, Pompey's troops became disoriented and were easily defeated when the Persians swept in.

Around 77 CE, the Roman naturalist Pliny the Elder cautioned against the toxic honeys from that region, calling them *meli maenomenon*—crazy honey. He correctly surmised that local rhododendron, azalea, and oleander species were responsible for its toxicity, but his hypothesis was not confirmed until chemists discovered plant-based grayanotoxins in honey in 1891.

Some scholars have suggested that mead spiked with mad honey may have played a part in the Dionysian Mysteries, the orgiastic rituals practiced in Ancient Greece and Rome, or in the prophetic trance state endowed upon the Oracle of Delphi.

In the mid-tenth century, once again on the south shores of the Black Sea, Olga of Kiev procured a decisive victory over Russian enemies with a poisoned gift of several tons of toxic honey. The Russians should have read up on Greek and Roman history or employed a taste tester: All 5,000 men were killed without much of a fight.

THE GURUNG HONEY HUNTERS OF NEPAL

In Nepal, a group of Gurung people known as the "honey hunters" have a time-honored but dangerous relationship with the honey—and its makers. The world's largest honeybee, the Himalayan honeybee, builds enormous hives, up to 5 feet (1.5 m) in diameter, high against the cliffs of the world's tallest mountain range.

The quest to harvest the honey is a serious endeavor, more akin to extreme sports than traditional beekeeping. Every spring and autumn, when the honey is at peak potency, a troop of male honey hunters trek high in the Himalayan peaks, where the rhododendrons are most plentiful. When they reach the cliff, they burn incense and say prayers, invoking the forest spirits to bless their harvest.

The hunters select one of the dozens of hives clinging like giant barnacles to the cliff. One group starts a fire at the base of the cliff, carefully directing the smoke toward the hive high above, and a second group secures a rope ladder at the top of the cliff. Then, a hunter gingerly descends into the gorge.

The bees do not give up their treasure easily. For several minutes, both the climber and his helpers must remain perfectly still to placate the furious swarm. Ignoring the constant stings, the hunter uses long bamboo rods to remove huge honeycombs from the hive and place them on suspended baskets, which are carefully lowered to the ground. Each hive can contain more than a hundred pounds (45 kg) of head-spinning honey.

When the troop returns to their village, a fevered celebration ensues. The locals enjoy a daily spoonful of the honey, believing it to have aphrodisiac and healing powers. But in today's global economy, mad honey has also become something of a niche cache crop, and the villagers sell most of the precious liquid to international buyers for a fine price.

In their communities, the honey hunters are heroes. With courage, cunning, and the wisdom of their ancestors, they brave the cliffs and return with the precious syrup. In spite of the dangers, the Gurung will keep scaling the cliffs and assailing the hives, just like their fathers and grandfathers before them. In this timeless drama of man versus nature, bitter conflict almost always leads to a sweet ending.

But rhododendron species containing grayanotoxins are not limited to the Black Sea region, and occurrences of contaminated honeys have popped up in other locales. In 1802, naturalist Benjamin Barton described how Pennsylvania beekeepers suffered from peculiar honey poisonings. And in 1875, a Confederate surgeon recounted how a number of soldiers fell ill after consuming local honeys, showing the same symptoms as Old World armies of prior eras. Poisonings have also occurred in the Pacific Northwest, mainly due to the predominance of mountain laurel, a poisonous plant in the same family as rhododendrons, but they're quite rare. Among large-scale honey producers, intoxication cases are almost unheard of. Modern production techniques, such as combining many honeys into one gigantic batch, have eliminated the risk.

MEDICINE AND RECREATION

Don't let its history in warfare fool you: Mad honey is much more than a poison. Prized as a precious intoxicant and rare medicine in the few communities where it is naturally produced, mad honey also fetches a high price on the global market. It is especially popular in Korea, Japan, and China, where many consumers consider mad honey a cure for erectile dysfunction.

In northern Turkey, where the mind-bending honey became the bane of Roman, Greek, and Russian troops throughout the centuries, *deli bal* has long been appreciated as a local delicacy. A spoonful may be mixed into a glass of milk for a sweet treat or added to an alcoholic beverage to heighten its inebriating effects. In the eighteenth century, Turkey exported two dozen tons of *deli bal* every year to Western Europe, where it was eagerly consumed by tavern patrons seeking more than the usual buzz.

Many Turks consider the honey a medicine, consuming it to treat diabetes, high blood pressure, and sexual dysfunction.

Today, many Turks consider the honey a medicine, consuming it to treat diabetes, high blood pressure, and sexual dysfunction. Turkish honey vendors still sell the sticky elixir, especially in the mountainous northeastern province Trabzon, but it's not well advertised. The locals are prudent enough to keep the potent stuff behind the counter, and only the most enterprising tourists are likely to discover it.

ACKNOWLEDGMENTS

I am indebted to many people for the creation of this book. To Jill Alexander, Julia Gaviria, and Mary Cassells, thank you for your deft editing hands—I am lucky to work with a skilled team who shares my creative vision. Many thanks to Marissa Giambrone, Holly Neel, and the Fair Winds art and design team for your incredible visual work. You brought these chapters to life. To all the Cave crew, especially Ross, Lee, Jonathan, Sanjay, and Dmitry, thank you for being my partners in exploration. There is nothing more valuable than a trusted friend when bushwhacking the frontiers of consciousness. To my parents, David and Patricia, thank you for stoking my creative fire from the very beginning. Some of my earliest memories are of making "books" from lined paper and crayons, and without your constant encouragement this book would not exist. To my brother, Shad, I'm grateful for your unwavering support through all the years. A big thanks to Quinn, for putting up with her dad's side project. And to Jill, my wife and partner in all things, thank you for your love and support—you made this project possible.

ABOUT THE AUTHOR

Cody Johnson lives in Boston with his wife, daughter, and two cats. He runs the popular blog PsychedelicFrontier.com, where he writes about the therapeutic, medicinal, and spiritual aspects of psychedelics. This is his first book.

Rätsch C. *The Encyclopedia of Psychoactive Plants: Ethnopharmacology and Its Applications*. Rochester, VT: Park Street Press; 2005.

Schultes RE, et al. *Plants of the Gods: Their Sacred, Healing, and Hallucinogenic Powers*. Rochester, VT: Healing Arts Press; 2001.

Stafford PG, Bigwood J. *Psychedelics Encyclopedia*. Berkeley, CA: Ronin Publishing; 1992.

Shulgin A, Shulgin A. *Pihkal: A Chemical Love Story*. Berkeley, CA: Transform Press; 1995.

2-C Family

Boal M. "The Agony & the Ecstasy of Alexander Shulgin." *Playboy*. 2004.

Benson T. "All 'Smiles': the history of the 2C designer drug class." *The Verge*. www.theverge.com/2015/7/15/8962743/all-smiles-the-history-of-the-2c-designer-drug-class. Published July 15, 2015.

Brown Ethan. "Professor X." *Wired Magazine*. September 1, 2002. www.wired.com/2002/09/professorx/. Published September 1, 2002.

Cohen D. *Freud on Coke*. Luton, UK: Andrews UK Ltd; 2011.

Mahavishnu. "Between Nothingness and Infinity: An Experience with 2C-B, 2C-C, 2C-E & 2C-I (exp85144)". Erowid.org. Jul 22, 2010. www.erowid.org/exp/85144.

Shulgin A. "2,5-dimethoxy-4-bromophenethylamine (2C-B)." Ask Dr. Shulgin Online. Center for Cognitive Liberty & Ethics. www.cognitiveliberty.org/shulgin/adsarchive/2cb.htm. Published Feb. 7, 2003.

5-MeO-DMT

Wade D, Weil A T. "Identity of a New World Psychoactive Toad." *Ancient Mesoamerica*. 1992;3(01):51–59. doi:10.1017/S0956536100002297.

Weil AT, Davis W. "Bufo alvarius: a potent hallucinogen of animal origin." *J Ethnopharmacol*. 1994,41(1 2):1–8. doi: 10.1016/0378-8741(94)90051-5.

Davis W. "Cultures at the far edge of the world." TED Talks. YouTube. https://youtu.be/bL7vK0pOvKI.

Grof S. *When the Impossible Happens: Adventures in Non-Ordinary Realities*. Boulder, CO: Sounds True; 2006.

Amanita muscaria

Feeney K. "Revisiting Wasson's Soma: exploring the effects of preparation on the chemistry of Amanita muscaria." *J Psychoactive Drugs*. 2010;42(4):499–506.

Feeney K. "The Significance of Pharmacological and Biological Indicators in Identifying Historical uses of Amanita muscaria." In: Rush J, ed. *Entheogens and the Development of Culture: The Anthropology and Neurobiology of Ecstatic Experience*. Berkeley, CA: North Atlantic Books; 2013:279–318.

Rogers R. *The Fungal Pharmacy: The Complete Guide to Medicinal Mushrooms and Lichens of North America*. Berkeley, CA: North Atlantic Books; 2011.

Riedlinger TJ. "Fly-Agaric Motifs in the Cú Chulaind Myth Cycle". Lecture given at the Mycomedia Millennium Conference as published on Erowid.org. Oct 29 1999, published by Erowid June 2005.

Miller RJ. *Drugged: The Science and Culture Behind Psychotropic Drugs*. New York, NY: Oxford University Press; 2014.

von Bibra BE, Ott J. *Plant Intoxicants: A Classic Text on the Use of Mind-Altering Plants*. Rochester, VT: Healing Arts Press; 1995.

von Strahlenberg PJ. *An Historico-geographical Description of the North and Eastern Parts of Europe and Asia, But More Particularly of Russia, Siberia, and Great Tartary*. London, England. J. Brotherton; 1738.

Ayahuasca

Levy A. "The Drug of Choice for the Age of Kale." *The New Yorker*. Sept. 12, 2016, www.newyorker.com/magazine/2016/09/12/the-ayahuasca-boom-in-the-u-s.

Metzner R. *Sacred Vine of Spirits: Ayahuasca*. Rochester, VT: Inner Traditions • Bear & Co; 2005.

Sanches RF, et al. "Antidepressant Effects of a Single Dose of Ayahuasca in Patients With Recurrent Depression: A SPECT Study." *J Clin Psychopharmacol*. 2016;36(1):77–81. doi: 10.1097/JCP.0000000000000436.

Halpern JH, et al. "Evidence of health and safety in American members of a religion who use a hallucinogenic sacrament." *Med Sci Monit*. 2008;14(8):SR15–22.

Grob CS, et al. "Human psychopharmacology of hoasca, a plant hallucinogen used in ritual context in Brazil." *J Nerv Ment Dis*. 1996;184(2):86–94.

Frecska E, et al. "The Therapeutic Potentials of Ayahuasca: Possible Effects against Various Diseases of Civilization." *Front Pharmacol*. 2016;7:35. doi: 10.3389/fphar.2016.00035.

Kandell J, Richard E. "Schultes, 86, Dies; Trailblazing Authority on Hallucinogenic Plants." *The New York Times*. Apr. 13, 2001. www.nytimes.com/2001/04/13/us/richard-e-schultes-86-dies-trailblazing-authority-on-hallucinogenic-plants.html.

Rudgley R. *The Encyclopedia of Psychoactive Substances*. London, England: Little, Brown & Company; 1998:26.

Cannabis

Abel EL. "Cannabis in the Ancient World." *Marihuana: the first twelve thousand years*. New York, NY: Plenum Publishing; 1980.

Russo EB, et al. "Phytochemical and genetic analyses of ancient cannabis from Central Asia." *J Exp Bot*. 2008;59(15):4171–4182. doi: 10.1093/jxb/ern260

Clarke R, Merlin M. *Cannabis: Evolution and Ethnobotany*. Oakland, CA: University of California Press; 2013.

Rätsch C. *Marijuana Medicine: A World Tour of the Healing and Visionary Powers of Cannabis*. Rochester, VT: Healing Arts Press; 2001.

Walton RP. "Description of the Hashish Experience." In: *Marihuana: America's New Drug Problem*. Philadelphia, Pennsylvania: J. B. Lippincott; 1938:86–114. www.cannabiscure.info/wp-content/uploads/2016/07/Description-of-the-Hashish-Experience-R.-P.-Walton-M.D.-1938.pdf.

Brown DT. *Cannabis: The Genus Cannabis*. UK: Harwood Academic Publishers; 1998.

Shi Y. "Medical marijuana policies and hospitalizations related to marijuana and opioid pain reliever." *Drug Alcohol Depend*. 2017;173:144–150. doi: https://doi.org/10.1016/j.drugalcdep.2017.01.006.

DiPT

Blom JD, Sommer IEC. *Hallucinations: Research and Practice*. New York, NY: Springer Publishing; 2012.

Shulgin AT, Carter MF. "N, N-Diisopropyltryptamine (DIPT) and 5-methoxy-N,N-diisopropyltryptamine (5-MeO-DIPT). Two orally active tryptamine analogs with CNS activity." *Commun Psychopharmacol*. 1980;4(5):363–9.

Acrimonius Funk. "Not Unlike a Velvety, Saucey, French Dish: An Experience with DiPT & Salvia divinorum (20x extract) (exp56700)." Erowid.org. Oct 19, 2006. www.erowid.org/exp/56700.

Kaleida. "Long Lost Novelty Restored: An Experience with DiPT (exp107477)." Erowid.org. Feb 23, 2016. www.erowid.org/exp/107477.

Azureskies. "An Economical Auditory Adventure: An Experience with DiPT (exp19709)." Erowid.org. Mar 15, 2007. www.erowid.org/exp/19709.

Anonymous. "Music Was Broken: An Experience with DiPT (exp14610)." Erowid.org. May 12, 2002. www.erowid.org/exp/14610.

Corey V, et al. "Psychoactive Substances." In: Blom JD, Sommer IEC, eds. *Hallucinations: Research and Practice*. New York, NY: Springer;2012:297–316.

DMT

Strassman R. *DMT: The Spirit Molecule, A Doctor's Revolutionary Research into the Biology of Near-Death and Mystical Experiences*. Rochester, VT: Park Street Press; 2000.

Szara S. "The Comparison of the Psychotic Effect of Tryptamine Derivatives with the Effects of Mescaline and LSD-25 in Self-Experiments." In: Garattini S, Ghetti V, eds. *Psychotropic Drugs*. New York, NY: Elsevier; 1957:460.

Leary T. *High Priest*. Berkeley, CA: Ronin Publishing; 1995:215 and 267.

McKenna TK, McKenna DJ. *The Invisible Landscape: Mind, Hallucinogens, and the I Ching*. San Francisco, CA: HarperCollins; 1993.

McKenna TK. "Nature Is the Center of the Mandala." Presented at: Shared Visions Bookstore, Berkeley, California, September 12, 1987. YouTube. https://youtu.be/5DfW_1gj8Zk.

McKenna TK. "Rap Dancing into the 3rd Millennium." Presented at: Starwood XIV Festival, Brushwood Folklore Center, Sherman, New York, July 19–24, 1994. YouTube. https://youtu.be/gMUqaFwmhG0.

McKenna TK, with Zuvuya. "Dream Matrix Telemetry." *Dream Matrix Telemetry*, Delirium Records, 1993.

Szára S. "DMT at fifty." *Neuropsychopharmacol Hung*. 2007;9(4):201–5.

DOx

Parker SF. *Conversations with Ken Kesey*. Jackson, MS: University Press of Mississippi; 2014.

Bureau of Drug Abuse Control. *Micro-Gram*. Nov 1967;1(1):1–2. www.erowid.org/library/periodicals/microgram/microgram_1967_11_v01n01.pdf.

Bureau of Narcotics and Dangerous Drugs. *Microgram*. May 1968;1(8):2. www.erowid.org/library/periodicals/microgram/microgram_1968_04_v01n07.pdf.

Yu B, et al. "Serotonin 5-Hydroxytryptamine2A Receptor Activation Suppresses Tumor Necrosis Factor-α-Induced Inflammation with Extraordinary Potency." *J Pharmacol Exp Ther*. 2008;327(2):316–323. doi:10.1124/jpet.108.143461.

Gabelt BT, et al. "Aqueous Humor Dynamics in Monkeys after Topical R-DOI." *Invest Ophthalmol Vis Sci*. 2005;46(12):4691–6. doi: 10.1167/iovs.05-0647.

Morris H, Smith A. "The Last Interview with Alexander Shulgin." VICE. May 1, 2010. www.vice.com/en_se/article/the-last-interview-with-alexander-shulgin-423-v17n5. Published May 1, 2010.

Dawks. "Is DOx any good?" Shroomery. July 4, 2013. www.shroomery.org/forums/showflat.php/Number/18555338. Published July 4, 2013.

Barfknecht CF, Nichols DE. "Potential psychotomimetics. Bromomethoxyamphetamines." *J. Med. Chem*. 1971 Apr;14(4)370–372.

Shulgin AT, et al. "4-Bromo-2,5-Dimethoxyphenylisopropylamine, a new centrally active amphetamine analog." *Pharmacology*. 1971;5(2)103–107.

DXM

Stanciu CN, et al. "Recreational use of dextromethorphan, 'Robotripping'-A brief review." *Am J Addict*. 2016 Aug;25(5):374–7. doi: 10.1111/ajad.12389.

Morris H, Wallach J. "From PCP to MXE: a comprehensive review of the non-medical use of dissociative drugs." *Drug Test Anal*. 2014 Jul-Aug;6(7-8):614–32. doi: 10.1002/dta.1620.

Anonymous. "My First Trip: An Experience with DXM (exp1883)." Erowid.org. Jun 16, 2000. www.erowid.org/exp/1883.

Addy P. "Facilitating Transpersonal Experiences with Dextromethorphan: Potential, Cautions, and Caveats." *Journal of Transpersonal Psychology*. 2007;39(1):1–22.

J Gelfer. "Towards a Sacramental Understanding of Dextromethorphan." *J Alt Spirit New Age Stud*. 2007 Sep;3:80–96.

DeRogatis J. "Let It Blurt, The Life and Times of Lester Bangs, America's Greatest Rock Critic." New York, NY: Broadway Books; 2000:37–38.

The Shadow. "DXM, a double-edged sword: An Experience with DXM (exp72)." Erowid.org. Oct 13, 2000. www.erowid.org/exp/72.

Thgilenin. "Beyond Words: An Experience with DXM (exp180)." Erowid.org. Aug 15, 2001. www.erowid.org/exp/180.

Xerxes. "Weird Memories On This Nervous Night: An Experience with DXM (exp6511)." Erowid.org. Feb 28, 2002. www.erowid.org/exp/6511.

White W. "The Dextromethorphan FAQ: Answers to Frequently Asked Questions about DXM." Erowid. org. www.erowid.org/chemicals/dxm/faq/dxx_faq.shtml.

Fish and Sea Sponges

de Haro L, Pommier P. "Hallucinatory Fish Poisoning (Ichthyoallyeinotoxism): Two Case Reports From the Western Mediterranean and Literature Review." *Clinical Toxicology.* 2006;44(2):185–8. https://doi.org/10.1080/15563650500514590.

Rudgley R. *The Encyclopedia of Psychoactive Substances.* London, England: Little, Brown & Company; 1998.

Bagnis R, et al. "Problems of Toxicants in Marine Food Products: 1. Marine biotoxins." *Bulletin of the World Health Organization.* 1970;42(1):69–88.

Kochanowska AJ, et al. "Secondary Metabolites from Three Florida Sponges with Antidepressant Activity." *J Nat Prod.* 2008 Feb;71(2):186–189. https://doi.org/10.1021/np070371u.

Mora C, et al. "How many species are there on Earth and in the ocean?" *PLoS Biology.* 2011 Aug;9(8):e1001127. https://doi.org/10.1371/journal.pbio.1001127.

Diers JA, et al. "Identification of antidepressant drug leads through the evaluation of marine natural products with neuropsychiatric

pharmacophores." *Pharmacol Biochem Behav.* 2008 Mar;89(1):46–53. https://doi.org/10.1016/j.pbb.2007.10.021.

Kochanowska-Karamyan AJ, Hamann MT. "Marine indole alkaloids: potential new drug leads for the control of depression and anxiety." *Chem Rev.* 2010 Aug 11;110(8):4489–4497. doi: 10.1021/cr900211p.

Morris H, Wallach J. "Sea DMT." VICE. March 26, 2013. www.vice.com/en_us/article/znqdve/sea-dmt-000481-v20n3. Published March 26, 2013.

Iboga

Ravalec V, et al. *Iboga: The Visionary Root of African Shamanism.* Rochester, VT: Park Street Press; 2004.

Lotsof HS. "Ibogaine in the treatment of chemical dependence disorders: clinical perspectives." *Bull. MAPS.* 1995;5:16–27.

Brown TK. "The use of ibogaine in the treatment of substance dependence." *Current Drug Abuse Reviews.* 2013;6(1):3–13. doi: 10.2174/15672050113109990001.

Smyth BP, et al. "Lapse and relapse following inpatient treatment of opiate dependence." *Ir Med J.* 2010;103(6):176–9.

Cappendijk SLT, Dzoljic MR. "Inhibitory effects of ibogaine on cocaine self-administration in rats." *Eur J Pharmacol.* 1993;241(2–3):261–5. https://doi.org/10.1016/0014-2999(93)90212-Z.

Rezvani AH, et al. "Attenuation of alcohol intake by ibogaine in three strains of alcohol-preferring rats." *Pharmacol Biochem Behav.* 1995;52(3):615–20. doi: 10.1016/0091-3057(95)00152-M.

Alper KR, et al. "Fatalities temporally associated with the ingestion of ibogaine." *J Forensic Sci.* 2012;57(2):398–412. doi: 10.1111/j.1556-4029.2011.02008.x.

Alper KR, et al. "The ibogaine medical subculture." *J Ethno pharmacol.* 2008;115(1):9–24. doi: 10.1016/j.jep.2007.08.034.

Alper KR, et al. "A Contemporary History of Ibogaine in the United States and Europe." The Alkaloids Chemistry and Biology. 2001;56:249–81.

Freedlander J. "Ibogaine: A Novel Anti-Addictive Compound—A Comprehensive Literature Review." *Journal of Drug Education and Awareness.* 2003;1:79–98.

Mutual_Ascendency. "Me and The Loon: An Experience with Tabernathe Iboga (Rootbark) (exp103942)." Erowid.org. Jan 2, 2016. www.erowid.org/exp/103942.

Ketamine

Garcia-Romeu A, et al. "Clinical applications of hallucinogens: A review." *Exp Clin Psychopharmacol.* 2016;24(4):229–268. doi: 10.1037/pha0000084.

Jansen K. *Ketamine: dreams and realities.* Sarasota, FL: Multidisciplinary Association for Psychedelic Studies; 2001.

Domino EF. "Taming the Ketamine Tiger." *Anesthesiology.* 2010;113:678–684. https://doi.org/10.1097/aln.0b013e3181ed09a2.

Hooper J. "John Lilly: Altered States." *Omni Magazine.* Jan 1983.

Morgan CJA, Curran HV. "Ketamine use: a review." *Addiction.* 2012;107(1):27–38. https://doi.org/10.1111/j.1360-0443.2011.03576.x.

Muetzelfeldt L, et al. "Journey through the K-hole: phenomenological aspects of ketamine use." *Drug Alcohol Depend.* 2008;95(3):219–29.

Krupitsky EM, Grinenko AY. "Ketamine Psychedelic Therapy (KPT): A Review of the Results of Ten Years of Research." *Journal of Psychoactive Drugs.* 1997;29:165–183. https://doi.org/10.1080/02791072.1997.10400185.

Niesters M, et al A. "Ketamine for chronic pain: risks and benefits." *Br J Clin Pharmacol.* 2014;77(2):357–67. doi: 10.1111/bcp.12094.

REFERENCES

LSD

Lee MA, Shlain B. *Acid Dreams, the Complete Social History of LSD: the CIA, the Sixties, and Beyond.* New York, NY: Grove Press; 1985.

Sewell RA, et al. "Response of cluster headache to psilocybin and LSD." *Neurology.* 2006;66(12):1920–2. doi: https://doi.org/10.1212/01.wln.0000219760.05466.43.

Carhart-Harris RL, et al. "Neural correlates of the LSD experience revealed by multimodal neuroimaging." *Proc Natl Acad Sci USA.* 2016;113(17):4853–8. doi:10.1073/pnas.1518377113.

Gasser P, et al. "Safety and efficacy of LSD-assisted psychotherapy for anxiety associated with life-threatening diseases." *J Nerv Ment Dis.* 2014;202(7):513–520. doi: 10.1097/NMD.0000000000000113.

Gasser P, et al. "LSD-assisted psychotherapy for anxiety associated with a life-threatening disease: a qualitative study of acute and sustained subjective effects." *J Psychopharmacol.* 2015;29(1):57–68. https://doi.org/10.1177/0269881114555249.

Grof S, et al. "LSD-assisted psychotherapy in patients with terminal cancer." *Int Pharmacopsychiatry.* 1973;8(3):129–144.

Jay Stevens. *Storming Heaven: LSD and the American Dream.* New York, NY: Grove Press; 1998: 208.

Krebs TS, Johansen PØ. "Lysergic acid diethylamide (LSD) for alcoholism: meta-analysis of randomized controlled trials." *J Psychopharmacol.* 2012;26(7):994–1002. doi: 10.1177/0269881112439253.

Dolder PC, et al. "LSD Acutely Impairs Fear Recognition and Enhances Emotional Empathy and Sociality." *Neuropsychopharmacology.* 2016 Oct;41(11):2638–2646. doi:10.1038/npp.2016.82.

Kaelen M, et al. "LSD enhances the emotional response to music." *Psychopharmacology.* 2015;232(19):3607–14. https://doi.org/10.1007/s00213-015-4014-y.

Hartogsohn I. "The American Trip: Set, Setting, and Psychedelics in 20th Century Psychology." *Bull. MAPS.* 2013;23(1):6–9.

Hofmann A. *LSD—My Problem Child.* Santa Cruz, CA: MAPS; 2009.

Wold R. "LSD and Psilocybin for Cluster Headaches: Preventing Pain, Saving Lives." *Bull. MAPS.* 2013;Special Edition:34–35.

Mad Honey

Williams C. *Medicinal Plants in Australia Volume 1: Bush Pharmacy.* Kenthurst, NSW: Rosenberg Publishing; 2010:223.

Lensky Y. *Bee Products: Properties, Applications, and Apitherapy.* Boston, MA: Springer; 1997.

Mayor A. "Mad Honey!" *Archaeology.* 1995;48(6):32–40.

Rätsch C. *Encyclopedia of Psychoactive Plants: Endopharmacology and Its Applications.* South Paris, ME: Park Street Press; 2005: 751–4.

Ott J. "The Delphic bee: Bees and toxic honeys as pointers to psychoactive and other medicinal plants." *Economic Botany.* 1998;52(3):260–266. https://doi.org/10.1007/BF02862143.

Caprara D. "Hunting for Hallucinogenic Honey in Nepal." VICE. September 13, 2016. www.vice.com/en_uk/article/hunting-for-hallucinogenic-honey-in-nepal-v23n6. Published September 13, 2016.

MDA

Mannich C, et al. "Über Oxyphenyl-alkylamine und Dioxyphenyl-alkylamine." *Ber Dtsc. Chem Ges.* 1910;43:189–197. doi:10.1002/cber.19100430126.

Baggott MJ, et al. "Investigating the Mechanisms of Hallucinogen-Induced Visions Using 3,4-Methylenedioxyamphetamine (MDA): A Randomized Controlled Trial in Humans." *PLoS ONE.* 2010;5(12):e14074. https://doi.org/10.1371/journal.pone.0014074.

Naranjo C, et al. "Evaluation of 3,4-Methylenedioxyamphetamine (MDA) as an adjunct to psychotherapy." *Med Pharmacol Exp Int J Exp Med.* 1967;17(4):359–64.

Stolaroff MJ. *The Secret Chief Revealed, Conversations with Leo Zeff, Pioneer in the Underground Psychedelic Psychotherapy Movement.* Santa Cruz, CA: MAPS; 2004.

Turek IS, et al. "Methylenedioxyamphetamine (MDA) subjective effects." *J Psychedelic Drugs.* 1974;6(1):7–14.

Weil AT. "The Love Drug." *J of Psychedelic Drugs.* 1976 Oct–Dec;8(4):335–337.

Associated Press. "$700,000 Awarded to Estate of Army Drug Test Victim." May 6, 1987. *Los Angeles Times.* http://articles.latimes.com/1987-05-06/news/mn-2486_1_chemical-warfare-agents. Published May 6, 1987.

Zinberg N. "Observations on the Phenomenology of Consciousness Change." *J of Psychedelic Drugs.* 1976;8(1):59–76.

MDMA

Substance Abuse and Mental Health Services Administration. *Results from the 2013 National Survey on Drug Use and Health: Summary of National Findings,* NSDUH Series H-48, HHS Publication No. (SMA) 14-4863. Rockville, MD: Substance Abuse and Mental Health Services Administration; 2014. Table 1.1B.

Nelson RJ. *An Introduction to Behavioral Endocrinology.* 3rd Ed. Sunderland, MA: Sinauer Associates; 2005:669–720.

Gasser P. "Psycholytic therapy with MDMA and LSD in Switzerland." *Newsletter of the Multidisciplinary Association for Psychedelic Studies.* 1994–5;5(3):3–7.

Johansen PØ, Krebs TS. "Psychedelics not linked to mental health problems or suicidal behavior: a population study." *J Psychopharmacol.* 2015;29(3):270–9. https://doi.org/10.1177/0269881114568039.

Greer G, Tolbert R. "Subjective Reports of the Effects of MDMA in a Clinical Setting." *J of Psychoactive Drugs.* 1986;18(4):319–327. https://doi.org/10.1080/02791072.1986.10472364.

REFERENCES

Garcia-Romeu A, et al. "Clinical applications of hallucinogens: A review." *Exp Clin Psychopharmacol.* 2016;24(4)229–268. https://doi.org/10.1037/pha0000084.

Doblin R, Rosenbaum, M. "Why MDMA Should Not Have Been Made Illegal." In: Inciardi JA, ed. *The Drug Legalization Debate* (2nd Ed.). London, England: Sage Publications, Inc.;1991.

Beck J, Rosenbaum M. "The Distribution of Ecstasy." In: *Pursuit of Ecstasy: The MDMA Experience.* Albany, NY: State University of New York Press; 1994.

St. John G. *Rave Culture and Religion.* London, England: Routledge; 2004:149.

Macie T. "I'm a veteran who overcame treatment-resistant PTSD after participating in a clinical study of MDMA-assisted psychotherapy. My name is Tony Macie— Ask me anything!" Reddit. April 16, 2014. www.reddit.com/r/IAmA/comments/23606g/im_a_veteran_who_overcame_treatmentresistant_ptsd/. Published April 16, 2014.

Freudenmann R W, et al. "The origin of MDMA (ecstasy) revisited: the true story reconstructed from the original documents." *Addiction.* 2006;101(9):1241–1245. https://doi.org/10.1111/j.1360-0443.2006.01511.x.

Morning Glory

Carod-Artal FJ. "Hallucinogenic drugs in pre-Columbian Mesoamerican cultures." *Neurologia.* 2015;30(1):42–9. https://doi.org/10.1016/j.nrleng.2011.07.010.

Niño-Maldonado AI, et al. "Efficacy and tolerability of intravenous methylergonovine in migraine female patients attending the emergency department: a pilot open-label study." *Head Face Med.* 2009;5:21. https://doi.org/10.1186/1746-160X-5-21.

Ott J. "The Delphic bee: Bees and toxic honeys as pointers to psychoactive and other medicinal plants." *Economic Botany.* 1998;52(3):260–266.

Koehler PJ, Tfelt-Hansen PC. "History of methysergide in migraine." *Cephalalgia.* 2008;28(11):1126–35. https://doi.org/10.1111/j.1468-2982.2008.01648.x.

Durán D. *Historia de las Indias de Nueva España.* México: Editorial Porrúa; 1967.

Stafford PG, Bigwood J. *Psychedelics Encyclopedia.* Berkeley, CA: Ronin Publishing; 1992:118–9.

Nitrous Oxide

Austin JH. *Zen and the Brain: Toward an Understanding of Meditation and Consciousness.* Cambridge MA: MIT Press; 2015:407–410.

Brown DJ. *The New Science of Psychedelics: At the Nexus of Culture, Consciousness, and Spirituality.* Rochester, VT: Park Street Press; 2013.

Gillman MA, Lichtigfeld FJ. "Analgesic nitrous oxide for alcohol withdrawal: a critical appraisal after 10 years' use." *Postgrad Med J.* 1990;66(777):543–6.

Gillman MA, Lichtigfeld FJ. "Enlarged double-blind randomised trial of benzodiazepines against psychotropic analgesic nitrous oxide for alcohol withdrawal." *Addict Behav.* 2004;29(6):1183–7.

Jacobsohn PH. "Horace Wells: discoverer of anesthesia." *Anesth Progr.* 1995;42(3–4):73–75.

James W. "Subjective Effects of Nitrous Oxide." *Mind.* 1882; Vol 7.

Nagele P, et al. "Nitrous oxide for treatment-resistant major depression: A proof-of-concept trial." *Biol Psychiatry.* 2015;78(1):10–18. http://dx.doi.org/10.1016/j.biopsych.2014.11.016.

Ojutkangas R, Gillman MA. "Psychotropic analgesic nitrous oxide for treating alcohol withdrawal in an outpatient setting." *Int J Neurosci.* 1994;76(1–2):35–9.

Tymoczko D. "The Nitrous Oxide Philosopher." *The Atlantic Monthly.* 1996 May;277(5):93–101. www.theatlantic.com/magazine/archive/1996/05/the-nitrous-oxide-philosopher/376581/.

Austin JH. *Zen and the Brain: Toward an Understanding of Meditation and Consciousness.* Cambridge MA: MIT Press; 2015:407–410.

Peyote

Huffman B. "Ken Kesey." *The Literary Encyclopedia.* First published 17 May 2002. www.litencyc.com/php/speople.php?rec=true&UID=4941.

Terry M, et al. "Lower Pecos and Coahuila Peyote: New Radiocarbon Dates." *Journal of Archaeological Science.* 2006;33(7):1017–1021. https://doi.org/10.1016/j.jas.2005.11.008.

Boyd CE. *The Rock Art of the Lower Pecos.* College Station, TX: Texas A & M University Press; 2003.

Boyd CE, Dering JP. "Medicinal and Hallucinogenic Plants Identified in the Sediments and the Pictographs of the Lower Pecos, Texas Archaic." *Antiquity.* 1996;70(268):256–275. doi: 10.1017/S0003598X00083265.

Stewart OC. *Peyote Religion.* Norman, OK: University of Oklahoma Press; 1987:24–42.

Huxley A. *The Doors of Perception.* UK: Chatto & Windus; 1954.

Gottlieb A. *Peyote and Other Psychoactive Cacti.* Berkeley, CA: Ronin Publishing; 1997.

Halpern JH, et al. "Psychological and Cognitive Effects of Long-Term Peyote Use Among Native Americans." *Biological Psychiatry.* 2005;58(8):624–631. https://doi.org/10.1016/j.biopsych.2005.06.038.

Psilocybin

Griffiths RR, et al. "Mystical-type experiences occasioned by psilocybin mediate the attribution of personal meaning and spiritual significance 14 months later." *J Psychopharmacol.* 2008;22(6):620–632. https://doi.org/10.1177/0269881108094300.

Lattin D. *The Harvard Psychedelic Club: How Timothy Leary, Ram Dass, Huston Smith, and Andrew Weil Killed the Fifties and Ushered in a New Age for America.* New York, NY: Harper Collins; 2011.

REFERENCES

Doblin R. "Dr. Leary's Concord Prison Experiment: A 34-Year Follow-up Study." *J Psychoactive Drugs*. 1998;30(4):419–26. https://doi.org/10.1080/02791072.1998.10399715.

Kingsborough, Lord. *Antiquities of Mexico*. (Ritos antiquos, vol. 9). London and New York;1848:17.

Samorini G. "The Oldest Representations of Hallucinogenic Mushrooms in the World (Sahara Desert, 9000–7000 B.P.)." *INTEGRATION Journal of Mind-moving Plants and Culture*, 1992;2&3:69–78.

Schleiffer H. *Sacred Narcotic Plants of the New World Indians*. New York, NY: Hafner Press; 1973:20–21.

Grob CS, et al. "Pilot study of psilocybin treatment for anxiety in patients with advanced-stage cancer." *Arch Gen Psychiatry*. 2011 Jan;68(1):71–8. doi: 10.1001/archgenpsychiatry.2010.116.

Moreno FA, et al. "Safety, tolerability, and efficacy of psilocybin in 9 patients with obsessive-compulsive disorder." *J Clin Psychiatry*. 2006;67(11):1735–40.

Cowen P. "Altered states: psilocybin for treatment-resistant depression." *The Lancet Psychiatry*. 2016;3(7):592–3. https://doi.org/10.1016/s2215-0366(16)30087-6.

Carhart-Harris RL, et al. "Psilocybin with psychological support for treatment-resistant depression: an open-label feasibility study." *The Lancet Psychiatry*. 2016;3(7):619–627. https://doi.org/10.1016/s2215-0366(16)30065-7.

Lebedev AV, et al. "Finding the self by losing the self: Neural correlates of ego-dissolution under psilocybin." *Human Brain Mapping*. 2015;36(6):2027–2038. https://doi.org/10.1002/hbm.22833.

Hendricks PS, et al. "Psilocybin, psychological distress, and suicidality." *J Psychopharmacol*. 2015 Sep;29(9):1041–1043. https://doi.org/10.1177/0269881115598338.

Hendricks PS, et al. "The relationships of classic psychedelic use with criminal behavior in the United States adult population." *J Psychopharmacol*. 2017;32(1):37–48. https://doi.org/10.1177/0269881117735685.

Schultes RE, Hofmann A, *Plants of the Gods: Their Sacred, Healing, and Hallucinogenic Powers*. Rochester, VT: Healing Arts Press; 1992:149.

Salvia

Valdés LJ III. The Early History of Salvia divinorum. *The Entheogen Review*. 2001;10(3):73–75.

Epling C, Játiva-M C. "A new species of Salvia from Mexico." *Botanical Museum Leaflets, Harvard University*. 1962;20(3):75–76.

Valdés LJ III, et al. "Ethnopharmacology of Ska María Pastora (Salvia Divinorum, Epling and Játiva-M.)." *J. Ethnopharmacology*. 1983;7:287–312.

Johnson JB. "The elements of Mazatec witchcraft." *Etnologiska Studier*. 1939;9:128–150.

Roth BL, et al. "Salvinorin A: A potent naturally occurring nonnitrogenous kappa opioid selective agonist." *Proc Natl Acad Sci U S A*. 2002;99(18):11934–9.

Ortega A, et al. "Salvinorin, a new trans-neoclerodane diterpene from Salvia divinorum (Labiatae)." *Journal of the Chemical Society Perkins Transactions 1*. 1982;0:2505–8.

San Pedro

Yerman D. *The Great Cacti: Ethnobotany & Biogeography*. Tuscon, AZ: University of Arizona Press; 2007:220–224.

Anderson EF. *The Cactus Family*. Portland, OR: Timber Press; 2001:45–49.

Hayes C. *Tripping: An Anthology of True-life Psychedelic Adventures*. Canada: Penguin Compass; 2001:328–331.

Davis EW. Sacred Plants of the San Pedro Cult. *Botanical Museum Leaflets, Harvard University*, 1983;29(4):367–386

Bussmann RW, Sharon D. "Traditional medicinal plant use in Northern Peru: tracking two thousand years of healing culture." *J Ethnobiol Ethnomed*. 2006;2:47.

Yopo

Kärkkäinen J, et al. "Urinary excretion of free bufotenin by psychiatric patients." *Biol Psychiatry*. 1988;24(4):441–446. https://doi.org/10.1016/0006-3223(88)90182-5.

Ott J. *Pharmacotheon:Entheogenic Drugs, Their Plant Sources and History*. Kennewick, WA: Natural Products Company; 1993:164–5.

Stafford PG, Bigwood J. *Psychedelics Encyclopedia*. Berkeley, CA: Ronin Publishing; 1992:309-331.

de Smet PAGM. "A multidisciplinary overview of intoxicating enema rituals in the western hemisphere." *J Eihnophormacol* 1983 Dec;9(2–3):129–66.

Altschul S. "The genus Anadenanthera in Amerindian cultures." Cambridge, MA: Botanical Museum, Harvard University; 1972.

Safford WE. "Identity of Cohoba, the Narcotic Snuff of Ancient Haiti." *Journal of the Washington Academy of Sciences*. 1916;6:547–562.

Emanuele E, et al. "Elevated urine levels of bufotenine in patients with autistic spectrum disorders and schizophrenia." *Neuro Endocrinol Lett*. 2010;31(1):117–1.

INDEX